MW00657517

To Kristy,

Laugh 'Til it Heals

Notes from the World's Funniest Cancer Mailbox

By
Christine K. Clifford

Illustrated by Jack Lindstrom

Don't forget to laugh!
Christine Clifford

Published by:-

Anshan Ltd
11a Little Mount Sion
Tunbridge Wells
Kent. TN1 1YS

Tel: +44 (0) 1892 557767
Fax: +44 (0) 1892 530358
e-mail: info@anshan.co.uk
web site: www.anshan.co.uk

ISBN: 978 1 848290 66 2

British Library Cataloguing in Publication Data

A catalogue record for this book is available from the British Library.

Editor: Tara Foss
Cover Design: Graham Rich
Cover and internal cartoons: Jack Lindstrom
Typeset by: Kerry Press Ltd, UK
Printed in the USA by:

DEDICATION:

To my sons Tim and Brooks for celebrating seventeen years of good health, good laughs, and good deeds with me since I was diagnosed with cancer. It's been an amazing ride with you by my side.

To all the members of The Cancer Club, who have brought me nothing but joy and laughter. God bless you all.

Laugh at Cancer

I saw a play at the National Theatre called "One Man, Two Guvnors" starring James Corden. I laughed 'till I hurt. I laughed so much, in fact, that I had to turn my back on the action in order to take another breath. Why was this pain so pleasurable? It's not masochism; it exists in its own right and although I couldn't make sense of it at the time, on reflection I deduced that this kind of pain must have an evolutionary advantage. I've looked after many cancer patients in my time and often cursed God for allowing such suffering. Yet after a moment's reflection, I reminded myself that without the nerve endings evolved to transmit pain, our species would have died out long ago. At the same time, I noticed that even in extremis my patients never lost their sense of humour. Putting it another way, a gift of a sense of humour, a sense of fun and a sense of the ridiculous, is the surest way to make friends and increase your popularity. Have you noticed in contrast how dictators and despots have had the sense of humour bypass operation? How else could they stomp around in those ridiculous uniforms and shirts? Such men are dangerous.

This wonderful book is the antidote to the slings and arrows of outrageous fortune and codifies the evolutionary advantage I was trying to grasp. Laugh at cancer, laugh with cancer, help cancer patients laugh; it's like the gentle rain from heaven and blesses the giver and receiver. It may not make you live longer, but it gives meaning to the remainder of your life and makes it worth getting up in the morning.

A man who was given only 6 months to live after a diagnosis of cancer wanted to make love to his wife 5 months and 30 days later. She declined saying, "It's all right for you, *I've* got to get up in the morning."

Professor Michael Baum
Prof. Emeritus of Surgery, University College, London.
Former President of the British Oncology Association
Former President of the European Breast Cancer Conference
Former Chairman of the Psycho-social committee of the National Cancer Research Institute
Prize winner: William McGuire prize, San Antonio Texas; Charles Gross prize, France; St Gallen prize Switzerland - the gold medal of the International College of Surgeons for his research into the treatment of breast cancer.

Author of *Breast Beating, A Personal Odyssey in the Quest for an Understanding Of Breast Cancer, The Meaning of Life, And Other Easy Questions*

Testimonials

"Christine has once more hit a home run with ***Laugh 'Til It Heals: Notes from the World's Funniest Cancer Mailbox***! The cancer survivors' testimonies about humorous events in their lives coupled with the insights of humor writers and practitioners about the power of humor, tied together with Christine's survivor wisdom is a well balanced read. I laughed, cried and then laughed again!"

–Dr. Ann Weeks, nurse family therapist and author of *She Laughs and the World Laughs With Her*

*****

"Christine Clifford does it again! In ***Laugh 'Til It Heals***, she shares hilarious stories that cancer survivors have provided her over the years. Many took me back to how gelotology (the study of humor) came to my rescue during and after my treatments for breast cancer. She also provides valuable resources on cancer-related organizations and therapeutic humor. The reader will thoroughly enjoy this collection of stories and the cartoons accompanying them."

– Jan Hasak, breast cancer survivor, speaker and author of *Mourning Has Broken: Reflections on Surviving Cancer* and *The Pebble Path: Returning Home from a Forest of Shadows*

*****

"Cancer is not funny. Still, funny things happen …and that is where the healing begins. Christine Clifford knows this well from her own experience with cancer. She also knows how to help others to find something funny in their not-so-funny situations. And she has done a masterful job of this in her latest book which invites readers to guffaw and get well."

-Allen Klein, author of *The Healing Power of Humor and Learning to Laugh When You Feel Like Crying*

*****

"Christine is right – laughter is the best medicine. Sometimes during my cancer treatment I roared at something I considered funny – but no one else did. Suspect it takes all sorts.

However, as soon as I saw Christine's cartoons, I knew they were just what I wanted to illustrate my book on Inflammatory Breast Cancer. Although IBC is no laughing matter, if we can have a joke, treatment goes much better. So I hope Christine will continue to make us laugh – and laugh at each other."

–Verité Reily Collins, author of *Inflammatory Breast Cancer: Explanation, Advice, Support*

Contents

Acknowledgements

"If anyone would tell you the shortest, surest way to happiness and all perfection, he must tell you to make it a rule to yourself to thank and praise God for everything that happens to you. For it is certain that whatever seeming calamity happens to you, if you thank and praise God for it, you turn it into a blessing."

– William Law

For me personally, cancer has been a gift. I certainly didn't think that on December 19, 1994 when I was told that I had cancer. But it changed my life in so many ways—wonderful ways, actually—that I have to say, I'm glad that I went through it to learn all the things about life that I've been exposed to because of cancer.

If someone had told me seventeen years ago, that I would create a company called The Cancer Club and spend all of my days laughing, I would have said they were crazy! But that's exactly what I've done. The cards, e-mails, letters, packages, and phone conversations that I've had with thousands of cancer patients has brought laughter into my life daily. How is it that all these people, facing the worst of the worst—cancer—have been able to find even the tiniest bit of humor? Because if we didn't laugh about it, we'd cry. And laughter feels *WAY* better than tears.

I want to thank my family: brothers Greg and James Meyer, and extraordinary step-mom Stephanie Meyer, and my "former family" John, Bette, and Bill Clifford who were beside me on my cancer journey.

I am deeply grateful to Shan and Andrew White, and Anshan Ltd. for believing in me and publishing this book and to Tara Foss for her editorial input.

To all my friends: Liz Robertson, Pat and Bucky Zimmerman, Virginia and Bob Carlson, Cheryl Sandeen, Kathy and Pat Lewis, Nancy Van Dyken, Parrel Caplan, Dawn and Jon Earl, Jean Golden, Lori Frank, Aija and Tom Meehan, Barb Greenberg, Gail Tilsner, Gregg Egginton, Jennifer

Shirley and Bruce Hazen, Tracy Stewart, Sue Bleecker, Bev Blize Nickerson, Marian and Dan O'Neil, Tom Schmidt, Jeff Lillemoe, Isaac Diaz, Jeff Evans, Gregory Brassil, Jim Greer, Jan Moore, Adele Brellenthin, Sally and Bill Hall, Barb Demos, C.J. Dube, Steve Schussler and Sunhi Ryan, Lauren and Merle Shapiro (and all the fabulous women of The Full Moon), Mary Barker, Mary Harlow, Mary McNutt, Michaelyn Born, Michael Collins, Randy Segal, Stacy Andresen, Vicki Rackner, Dr. Burt Schwartz, Dr. Tae Kim, Dr. Margit Bretzke, the staff at Minnesota Oncology Hematology, Margie and Mark Sborov, and all the women of Divorcing Divas: Susan Garfield, Karen Stafford, Jessie Welf, Joelle Pink, Michelle Palmer, Kim Rauser, Sharon Hall, Linda Margl, Alison Nelson, Melinda Bonk, Christina Boyd, Barbara Bencini, Jeanne Rosengren, Gary Hansen, Linda Olup, Morrie Wagner, Diana Pierce, Deb Hopp, Carla Beaurline, Lisa Wohlfert, Kristin Harper, and all of our sponsors, vendors, volunteers, and attendees of our events. Thank you for your support!

But most of all, I want to thank the vision and memory of my mom, Mary Christine Meyer, for reminding me every day how lucky I am to be alive. I miss you, Mom, and know one day, I shall see you again.

Introduction

"Laughter reaches a place no medicine can touch: the soul."

– Christine Clifford

It can split your sides, keep you in stitches, or make you fling milk out of your nose.

You can do it until you cry, until it makes you lose your breath, or God forbid, you actually wet your pants.

In short, laughter would seem to be more dangerous than driving with my son Brooks, an activity so hazardous that those insurance executives reading his application for auto insurance chortle so loudly that the people in their offices upstairs can hear it.

Like those split-sided executives, you really can laugh until it hurts. So it seems that when you are confronted with the words you dread most from a doctor, laughing is, if not the last thing you need, the last thing you may feel like doing.

But trust me, as a woman who stared at the Grinning Reaper and made fun of his silly outfit:

Laughter *is* very good medicine. It saved something at least as important as my life: my spirit. And it can save yours, too.

Years ago I wrote books about how laughter healed me, and for years following, thousands of people sent me letters about how laughter helped them, too. They sent those letters to The Cancer Club, which now owns the title of "The World's Funniest Cancer Mailbox."

These are their stories. I recommend that you avoid drinking milk before you read them.

Chapter 1
When the Joke's on You

WARNING: Humor may be hazardous to your illness ...

– Christine Clifford

A few years after completing my cancer treatments, I broke one of my toes (the same one, mind you) three times. The first time, I was angry at my clumsiness (I tripped over my son's hockey skates in the middle of July). The second time, I was astounded at my stupidity, knowing that I had developed chemotherapy-induced osteoporosis. But the third time, I simply had to laugh. It was God's way of telling me I needed some new material.

Finding the humor in life's challenges and particularly as it relates to the cancer experience, is what helps us get through the day; it reminds us of life's absurdities, and provides relief from the stress and strain of our treatments. If you've been feeling sad or low, you've come to the right place.

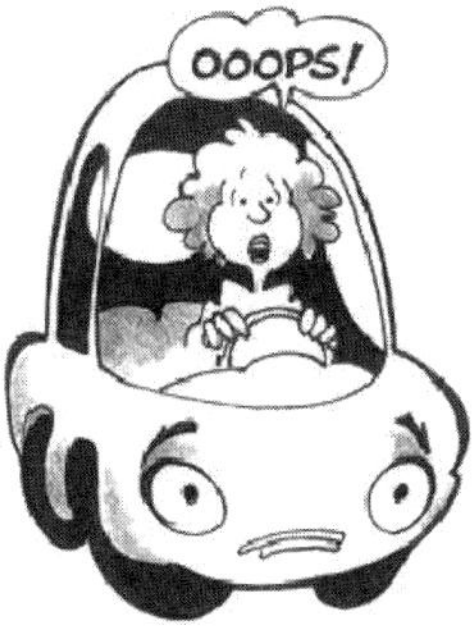

I read somewhere once, "When everything's coming your way, you're in the wrong lane." Sometimes things just don't go according to plan.

As a seventeen-year survivor, I am often asked what would be the #1 thing that I feel contributed to my success as a survivor. While there have been many, many things, I am confident that #1—for me—was finding something to focus on that took my mind off my cancer, and gave me something new and exciting to look forward to.

In the beginning, that focus may be as simple as getting fresh flowers on your table every day, or being able to take a walk outdoors to feel the fresh air on our faces. It may be to get back to work after surgery, or to make an extended trip to see a loved one or dear friend.

As time goes by, our focus may change and may be based on doing that "something" in your life that you've always wanted to do. I know for me, that focus became The Cancer Club and searching for humor every day, which would not only help me, but help all of you as well.

Patty Wooten, RN, President of Jest for the Health of It, author, speaker, cancer survivor, and 2002 recipient of the "Lifetime Achievement Award" from the Association for Applied and Therapeutic Humor, has this to say about using humor to get through a cancer experience:

Managing cancer is serious business. The treatments are toxic, the stakes are high, and the situations with which a patient must cope are often treacherous. Why would anyone want to laugh under these circumstances?

Because laughter and humor can help you get past the unpleasant, manage the unbearable, and cope with the unexpected.

Humor is a perpetual event. It is a way of looking at things. No two people see things the same way, so there is a wide range of what can be defined as humorous. Men's perceptions of what is funny tend to be different than women's. With regard to illness, humor is the ability to perceive and find something funny in the face of adversity. Sometimes, humor provides us with a way to distance ourselves just enough from a troublesome experience to be able to tolerate it.

Laughter is a behavioral event. It is a physical response to humor that can engage the entire body and involve most of the major muscle groups. The extent to which your body changes is related, in part, to how comfortable you feel with losing control. When you first recognize that something is funny, your breathing pattern changes, then you develop a smirk which turns into a smile and is followed by a grin. Next, you begin to make noises, ranging from controlled snickers, escaped chortles and giggles to cackles, hoots, and guffaws. As the noise grows louder, you may begin to sway back and forth, slap your knees, stomp your feet or jab your elbow into someone nearby. As your laughter peaks, tears may begin to flow freely. When you are finished laughing, you may feel weak and exhausted for a while. Laughter serves as a safety valve to release worries, relax, and let go.

Janet Henry had breast cancer. After her mastectomy, she had chemotherapy. So, first she lost her breast and then she lost her hair. But she never lost her sense of humor. Her humor gave her courage and hope. She wrote a series of poems. Here's one of my favorites:

The Nightly Ritual

I prop my wig up on the dresser
And tuck my prosthesis beneath
And I thank God; I still go to bed
With my man and my very own teeth.

Remember: if you can laugh at it, you can live with it.

Here's how some of our Cancer Club members decided to live … and focus:

Dear Cancer Club,

As my first morning at the radiation treatment center progressed, I was measured for my protective lead alloy molds, experienced a simulation run-through, and had a Computerized Tomography scan. I tried valiantly to absorb the new terminology and technology and to lie perfectly still during the various procedures.

I forgot about my husband's Valentine's Day request, until I noticed that the right side of my chest had acquired an array of ugly, black felt-tip pen markings. The thirty-something male technician was placing wide strips of transparent tape over the marks while explaining, "These markings are made with permanent marker, but I'm putting tape over them to make sure they don't wash off before your next appointment."

He must have read the dismay in my eyes, because he continued, "You don't have a problem with that, do you?"

Feeling a bit vulnerable and foolish lying on the table, bare from the waist up except for my black marks and transparent tape strips, I blurted out my husband's Valentine's Day request, "If this was any day but Valentine's Day, I wouldn't care. But I don't think my husband had black marks and tape strips in mind when he said he hoped I'd wear my transparent negligee tonight."

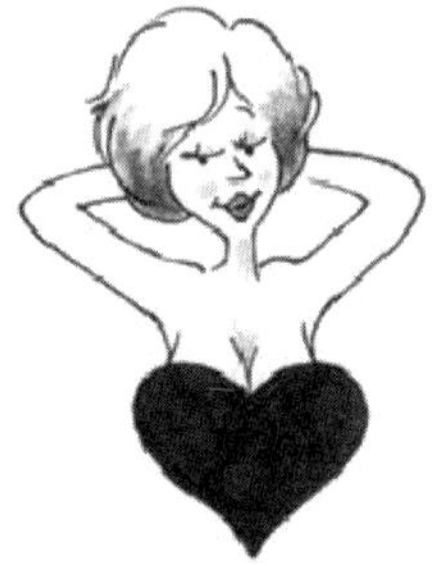

Blushing a rosier rose than my soon-to-be worn negligee, the technician walked to a cabinet and returned with a handful of small packets. Handing them to me, he said with a wink, "It's too long to expect you to keep these marks intact anyway. Just peel the tape off and use these cleaning pads to remove the marks. I'll re-mark you when you come in for your next appointment."

As I left the room, he smiled and said, "You two have a great Valentine's Day!"

** Sharon Callister*
** Cannon Falls, MN*

* * * * *

Dear Cancer Club,

I'm not kidding. I received my breast cancer diagnosis on April Fool's Day.

Prior to having a bone scan/MRI, I was given a liquid to drink. I was told, however, that for some people, it is a very powerful diuretic. So, as I was crossing the street to the hospital, it was becoming increasingly apparent that I needed to find a bathroom. Quickly.

As I was entering the lobby of the Duke Medical Center, the you-know-what hit the fan. I was so horrified, I accosted the first white lab-coated female I could find, and very tensely, asked where the nearest restroom was.

She took one look at my face and asked, "What was the matter?" I told her that I was ******** all over the place!! Without batting an eye, she got right behind me, and we shuffled to the bathroom, where she left me to go find a set of scrubs.

As I was standing at the sink, washing out my pants (which, obviously, I was no longer wearing), I looked in the mirror and caught a glimpse of myself—complete with drainage tube from my mastectomy hanging out—just as an innocent bystander walked in to use the facilities.

I looked at myself, looked at her, back at myself, and just started laughing. At this point, dignity was totally out the window, and I just thought, "Well, THIS day isn't going to get any worse!"

As I made the rounds of appointments that day, I was injected with something and told that it causes some people to have the sensation that they need to urinate, but was assured that it wouldn't happen. Again, I thought it was hilarious. Urinate! That's nothing!

** Betty Thompson*
** Chapel Hill, NC*

* * * * *

Dear Cancer Club,

Surgery for acinic cell carcinoma of the parotid gland (salivary gland cancer) left me with an 8" incision along my neck, held together with metal staples. I went to sleep as Ms. McCutcheon and woke up Ms. McFrankenstein. My ex-boyfriend offered me a couple of bolts to complete the look. (You can tell why he's an ex.) Since then, I've had a remarkable recovery. I owe my life to my surgeon, whom I've since nominated for a knighthood.

I took about three weeks off work to recover from surgery and didn't start radiation until nearly eight weeks later. Given that I was only 34 years old and healthy (cancer aside), I was determined to keep working throughout the five weeks of radiation therapy. This arrogance was challenged after day two of treatments, when during a conference call at the office, I suddenly lost 90% of the moisture in my mouth.

Lest you have any doubt, saliva is essential to conversation. You never appreciate the value of saliva until the moment you have none.

With me, it was like a form of torture. Thank God I happened to have a bottle of water on my desk or I might have had to use sign language to tell my colleague to finish the call on my behalf. I can laugh about this now, and actually laughed pretty soon after it happened. I chalked it up to yet another learning experience: always have a bottle of water handy during treatment. I'm convinced I'll be carrying around a water bottle—much like a security blanket—until my salivary glands are back to normal.

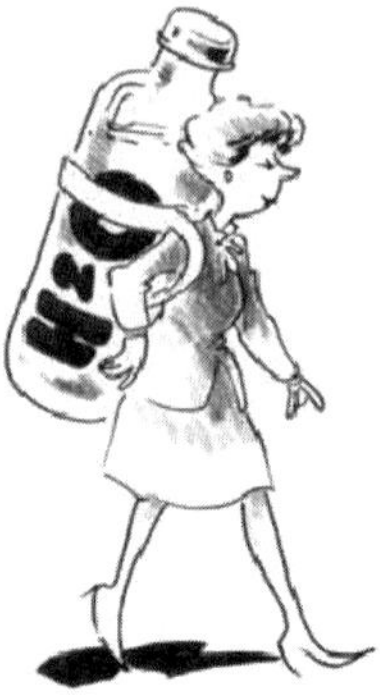

*** Ann McCutcheon**
*** Vancouver, British Columbia, Canada**

* * * * *

Dear Cancer Club,

When I went for my first chemo treatment, I had to fill out a health questionnaire about pre-existing problems, such as heart disease, kidney disease, lung disease and so on. After completing the form, the nurse said to the other staff nurses, "Look at this: nothing checked. She is the healthiest person with cancer we've had in a long time!"

Made me feel good. NOT!

I had to cross a parking lot during a wind storm, and I was concerned about my wig staying on. It did stay on, but I told my friend Chris how upset I would have been if it flew off in front of my co-workers.

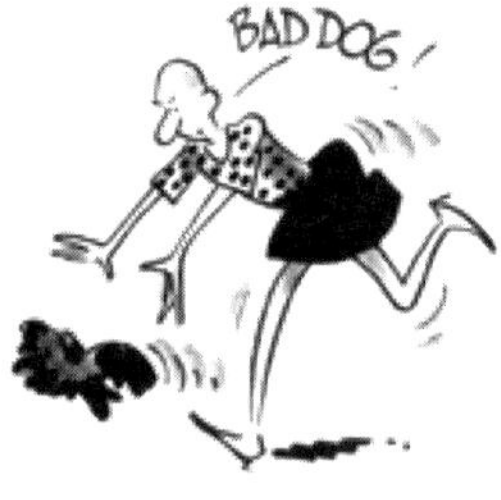

Chris suggested I should run after it, yelling, "Fluffy! Get back here! Bad dog!"

She made me laugh. So now my wig's name is Fluffy. I will tell my husband that tonight Fluffy is getting a bath.

*** Leslie Warren**
*** Toronto, OH**

Dear Cancer Club,

I went to have lunch with several former co-workers at a restaurant in Plano, Texas. This was the first time I'd had lunch with them since I started chemo for ovarian cancer.

I was dressed in nice business clothes and wearing my best wig. As I got out of my car, which was parked by the curb outside the restaurant, a gust of wind came around the building and caught my wig!

It flew off my head and rolled like a Texas tumbleweed across the parking lot, past rows of cars. I chased after it. Each time I stopped to pick it up, the wind caught it again and blew it even farther. I finally stomped on it to hold it down so that I could pick it up. It had blown across two driving lanes in the parking lots and past three rows of cars!

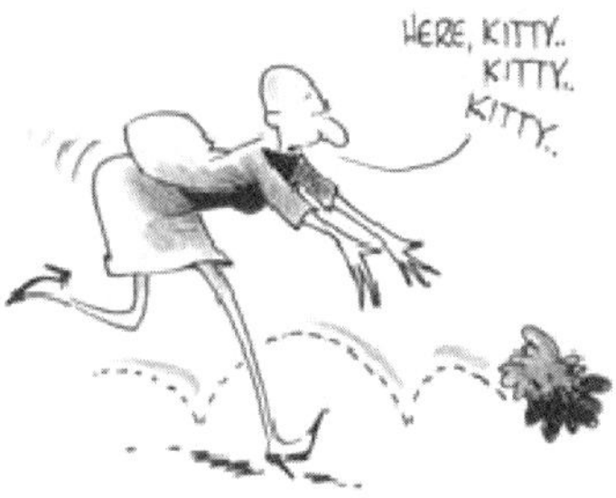

I scooped it up, shook it good to put the curls back in place and placed it on my bald, shiny head. Walking back across the parking lot, I wondered who had seen me. I was embarrassed at first and checked my appearance in the mirror, but when I thought about how funny I must have looked while chasing that rolling varmint, I laughed until my sides hurt!

** Mildred Pittman*
** Garland, TX*

* * * * *

Dear Cancer Club,

Shortly after 9/11, I had to fly from Portland, OR to a small city on business. I carry a badge in my purse, but I am not a cop. It is a seven point badge which could easily be a "throwing star," quite a dangerous object in the right (or wrong) hands. I often pass through this little airport, and security people there always catch it. This time, as I was going through the process on the return flight to Portland, I had the opportunity to have a short adventure, and I couldn't pass it up. I put my purse, briefcase and pager on the X-ray belt and walked through the metal detector. Even though I didn't activate it, they asked me to step aside so a sweet, little lady of about 65 could wave the handheld scanner over me. I stood there with my arms straight out from my sides, while she waved it all around me. Once the scanning is done, the sweet thing tells me she has to do a pat search. She starts rubbing the back of her hand across my outstretched arms, up and down my legs and across my chest before she asks me to turn around so she could repeat the same process.

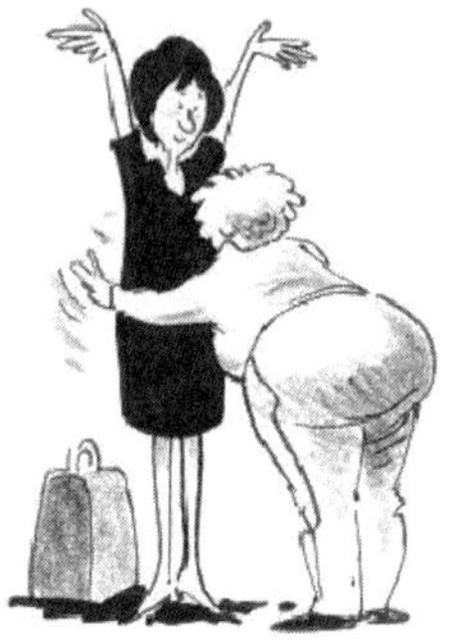

After all of this searching "stuff," I went over to the man holding my purse for me. He asked if I minded if he looked. I told him the item he was looking for was in the outside pocket of the purse, and would he mind if I got it out for him. He allowed me to do so. Once the badge was in his hands, he yells down the way to his buddies on the X-ray machine who saw it, "She's a cop! Look at this! It's a gold badge from the State of Oregon."

Of course, all the fellas had to come see it.

After all this high drama, the sweet little lady comes over to me and says, "Since you're a cop, tell me: was the pat search okay?" I couldn't help myself. I leaned close to her and whispered, "It was fine. But did you notice I had a phony breast?"

There was a brief gasp, and she just looked at me as her face turned red. I couldn't leave her like that, so I said, "So, I guess I got a high quality breast if you didn't notice it was fake, huh?" I was grinning like a fool, and she finally got into it and laughed a little.

Then she laughed a lot, and her male helpers wanted to know what they missed. I collected my belongings and strolled away, while she giggled and they badgered her to share the joke. I don't know if she shared the joke, and I don't really care if she did. It was funny, and I needed a laugh. Sometimes the joke is on you!

It's true: my hair has begun to return. And that is a very good thing for obvious reasons. But there are some not so obvious reasons why this is a very good thing. I am looking forward to the day when I have hairs in my nose again. Why?

So my nostrils don't stick together when I wipe my nose. Most people don't realize this is a concern. But to those of us who have been through the joys of chemo, we know. Those little hairs in each nostril were very thoughtfully designed because they are just enough to interrupt the sticking-together-process. And when your nose sticks together as you're making a point during a business meeting, well … you just lose a little bit of your thunder, don't you think?

*** Les S. Dolecal**
*** Stayton, OR**

* * * * *

Dear Cancer Club,

I have colon cancer and wear a colostomy bag. One Sunday, during service, it started to fill up very quickly, so I whispered to my husband, "I'll be right back."

Being the only one in the restroom, I decided that before I sat down on the loo, I would take off my wig because my head itched. I tossed it onto the back of the toilet, only to have it fall in! I quickly pulled it out, and was thankful that I hadn't done my "thing" yet. But I was upset because there was no way out of it unless I either walked back into the service bald, or put my wig back on.

Needless to say, I decided wearing a wet wig wasn't as bad even as a wig that had fallen into the loo. That was just one of my "no hair" days!

*** Wendy Kilmer**
*** White Cloud, MI**

Dear Cancer Club,

My funny episode was a day at work. I own a small shop with flags, banners, and windsocks. I was taking a windsock off the floor for a customer when another sock hanging from a battery-operated spinner got caught in my wig, spinning and spinning until it was wrapped up in all my plastic hair!

I had to remove my wig, take down the spinner from the ceiling, and carefully remove the metal. I thought I was going to wet my pants, I was laughing so hard! The customer ignored the entire thing. Ovarian cancer. Cancer free eight months and counting!

** Terri Horne*
** Cincinatti, OH*

* * * * *

Dear Cancer Club,

About four months after my surgery, I attended a support group meeting where they displayed prostheses. One woman spoke up and said she simply used a shoulder pad in her bra and that helped a lot. I liked that idea.

The following Saturday night I was invited to a friend's house and thought this would be the perfect time to try the shoulder pad. We played board games, watched a movie, and then moved to the table to play cards. On his way over to the table, Jim leaned over to the floor and said, "Did someone lose a shoulder pad?" I was laughing so hard that I had to tell them where it came from. Now I use safety pins.

** Gwen Myers*
** Columbus, OH*

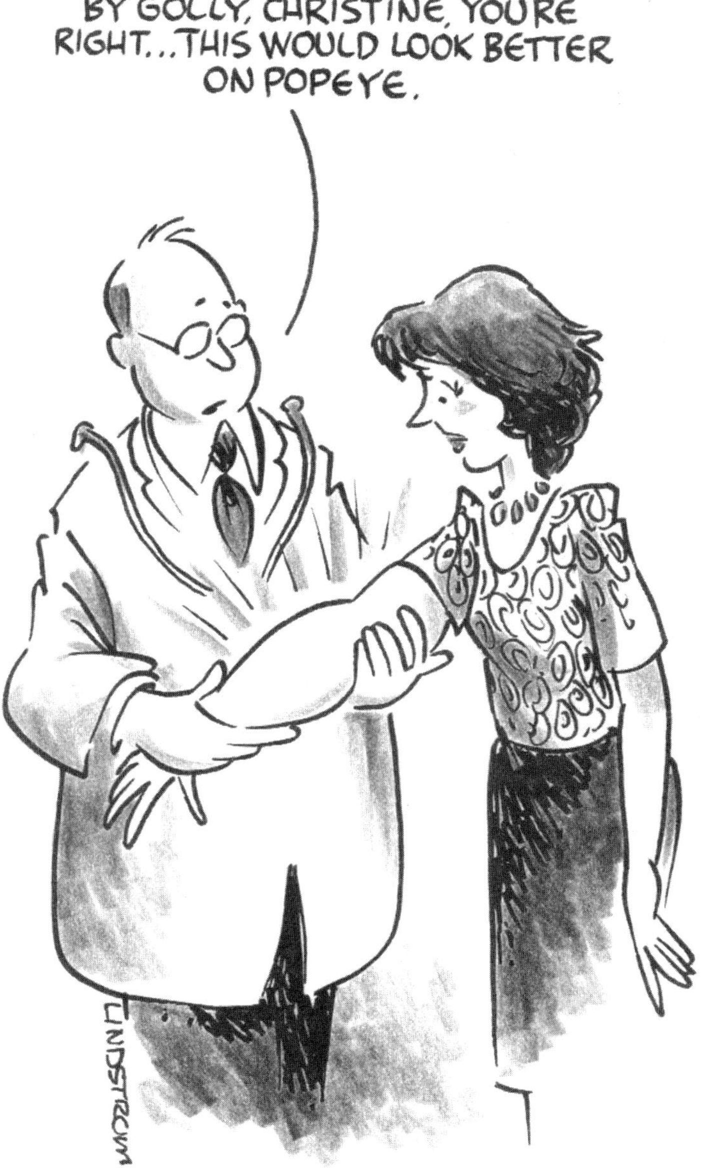
BY GOLLY, CHRISTINE, YOU'RE RIGHT...THIS WOULD LOOK BETTER ON POPEYE.
LINDSTROM

Chapter 2: Doctor, You've Got Me in Stitches!

"The purpose of the doctor is to entertain the patient while the disease takes its course."

– Voltaire

I have been truly blessed with an exceptional group of doctors. I really got to put Voltaire's theory to the test a few years ago. After nine-plus years of being a cancer survivor, I decided (at the urging of my beloved oncologist Dr. Burt Schwartz) to find out if I was, as we suspected, a carrier of the BRCA1 gene that causes hereditary breast cancer. After all, my mother had passed away at the age of 42 from the disease, and my sister (four years younger than me), had already tested positive.

Sure enough, I was one of the "lucky ones." Now I learned that as a carrier of the gene, I was also at more than 55% increased risk of developing ovarian cancer. So I took the bull by the horns and underwent an elective radical hysterectomy.

I share this story with you for two reasons. Number One: aren't we all blessed to be living in a world so advanced in medicine and technology that we can actually *change* the course of our futures? New drugs, new protocols, new surgeries are available to us every day.

But Number Two: I feel particularly blessed to have found yet another caring, thoughtful, educated, and *funny* physician to add to my already long list of specialists. Dr. Matthew Boente, head of the Division of Gynecologic Oncology at the University of Minnesota, had me laughing even as I was being wheeled into surgery (maybe it was the laughing gas, who knows?). And my point is this: there are wonderful, empathetic physicians out there who really care about us as human beings.

Here is the perspective from Dr. Clifford Kuhn, a psychiatrist *and* a comedian, and Professor of Psychiatry at the University of Louisville School of Medicine.

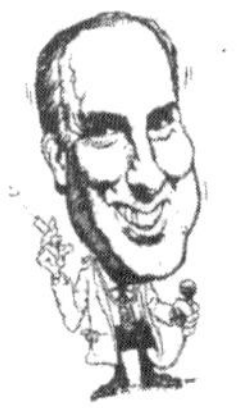

Lisa was fifteen years old when she sought my help. It had been six weeks since she learned that the pain in her leg was a malignant tumor. Her doctors told her she had about six months to live. She hastened to inform me that, with my help, she was going to outlast that prediction. And so she did.

For the next five years, until her death at age twenty, Lisa and I worked together to enhance her healing resources. They were five rollicking years, filled with many special experiences for her—graduating from high school, attending college, falling in love, becoming engaged, getting married, and spending a magical honeymoon in Hawaii. If you think Lisa got cheated in life, you simply did not know her. She packed more living into 20 years than most of us will in four times that span. During the years we were together, Lisa taught me many things. The most important lesson was to laugh during serious moments.

You see, I had always "approved" of laughter, but only in its place and time, which was after all responsibilities had been fulfilled. Lisa held that if we waited to meet my criteria, we might never laugh. She thought laughter's place was everywhere, and its time, any time. This was not an effort at denial or avoidance. Lisa took her cancer very seriously.

Instead, it was an example of a remarkable young person who chose to live the years she was given by transcending her adversities. I use the term "transcendence" to describe Lisa's accomplishments because I watched her virtually rise above her limitations. Transcendence is very different from avoidance. In avoidance, we ignore, deny, or otherwise skirt the unwanted truth. In transcending it, we acknowledge the pain, but maintain a perspective that prevents it from disabling us.

What was Lisa's secret? She respected her sense of humor and was willing to trust it. She understood what humor was and what it was not. In a term paper written for her English composition course, Lisa put it this way:

"... a sense of humor goes beyond the ability to tell an amusing anecdote and includes a capacity to see the positive aspects of otherwise adverse situations. I use my own sense of humor to help me remain sane through the difficult times in my battle with cancer."

As you know, some things in life are not negotiable. Certain losses cannot be resolved or compensated. We either rise above them or become mired in resentment and despair.

Quality of life is the issue here. Lisa demonstrated that an opportunistic sense of humor can lift us over our fear and pain, if we are willing. We may be victims of circumstance, but, with humor, we can be masters of response.

* * * * *

Dr. Bernie Siegel, a beloved and inspiring figure to all cancer patients, once said, "Show me a patient who is able to laugh and play, who enjoys living, and I'll show you someone who is going to live longer."

Here are some stories from experiences with doctors who tickled our funny bones:

Dear Cancer Club,

When in an examining room at a hospital emergency room, my friend—a double mastectomy patient—was being examined by a young intern. While removing her gown and checking her heart, making small talk, the doctor asked my friend if she had ever been in a hospital before.

She quite candidly said to the doctor, "No, I did this to myself."

Needless to say, the doctor was quite embarrassed when he realized what he had just said. Hopefully this will bring some humor into a life or two, or maybe more.

**** Dianne Garrett***
**** Brodrick House, Marysville, OH***

Dear Cancer Club,

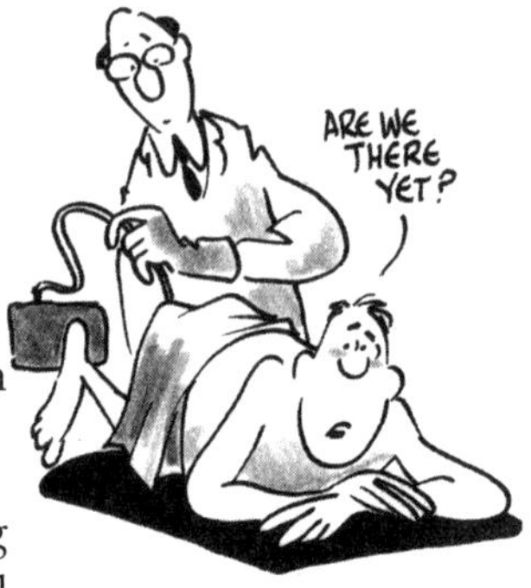

Sometimes I worry about my doctor. Recently, he rushed his first eight patients to the hospital in an ambulance. Then he found out his stethoscope was broken.

He will give me a physical exam; then put on plastic gloves to shake my hand.

One time, he really made me nervous by giving me a very unusual prescription: Two aspirin and a plane trip to Lourdes.

He's the type who likes to break things to you gently. I said, "Doc, do I have anything serious?" He said, "Only if you have plans for next year."

Another time I said, "Doc, what can you give me for my liver?" He said, "How about a pound of onions?"

I went to see him last winter with chills and fever. I said, "Doc, what would you call this?" He said, "Do you want the technical term?" I said, "Of course I do." He said, "Shake and bake."

I have learned one thing about my doctor. After an exam, a long, thoughtful, confident nod means: "Your guess is as good as mine."

Two things upset me about going to my doctor's office. When they leave the door ajar—and when they hand you one.

Now I lay me down to sleep
I pray the Lord my soul to keep.
If I should die before dawn's crack,
Tell my doctor, "He's a no-good quack!"

** Walter H. Perkins*
** Ocean, NJ*

Dear Cancer Club,

Convalescence

The breast it was malignant,
And so they took it off,
And now I hold a pillow
Every time I have to cough.

I thought that I was mending,
But things turned even worse,
I got a staph infection,
The surgical patient's curse.

Privacy and dignity
Belong to days gone by,
I try to keep on laughing,
'Cause otherwise, I'd cry.

My right arm it is painful,
There's a tube stuck in my left,
It shouldn't be surprising
That I'm feeling so bereft.

I sit here mesmerized
By the drip of my IV line,
And hope and pray the drugs in there
Will help me to feel fine.

I'm afraid I'm just not good
At the business of being ill,
But I know that I'll be really sick,
When I get the doctor's bill!

** Rose A. Sodergren*
** Sun City, AZ*

Dear Cancer Club,

As a sales representative for a pharmaceutical company, I come into contact with hundreds of cancer patients. One day, during the holidays, a patient turned to me and said, "I've lost a breast, and I only have one eye. What do you think I should ask for, for Christmas?!"

*** Diane Hall**
*** Columbia, SC**

* * * * *

Dear Cancer Club,

Mastectomy Blues

I fear I have contracted
A case of mastectomy blues.
It gives a whole new meaning
To keeping "abreast of the news."

I've been poked, and I've been prodded,
I've been stitched, and I've been drained.
At times I wanted to scream,
But so far I have refrained.

Doctor says I'm not to use
My right arm much at all,
Which makes things mighty awkward
When I answer Nature's call.

All toilet paper holders
Are on the right side of the "can,"
A major inconvenience
No doubt, thought of by a man.

When everything is healed,
I'll start all this again.
I'm going to get re-built
So maybe I'll be a "ten."

I hope my plastic surgeon
Isn't some dumb turkey,
Because I'm deadly serious
When I say that I want "perky!"

***Rose A. Sodergren**
©October, 2002
Sun City, AZ

* * * * *

Dear Cancer Club,

I'm an odd duck. I knew how to whistle when I was still in my baby bed. Unfortunately, there was no demand for a whistling baby, child, teenager, or adult—until I underwent treatment for a very aggressive form of breast cancer four years ago.

Unbeknownst to me, the staff in the radiation department could hear every sound in the room where I changed in preparation for my daily "zapping." After finishing a rousing rendition of "Oh, What a Beautiful Morning," I discovered that I had a fan club standing outside the door!

It seemed that a new and different (mostly male) technician gave each treatment. So on my last day, I wasn't too surprised when one of the guys said he had fourteen friends waiting outside to observe. I laughingly told him that they might as well come in but that they must all take responsibility for my new career as a speaker. I didn't bat an eyelash (I didn't have any to bat anyway!).

I just smiled sweetly and said, "Since almost all the men in this county have seen me without my blouse, my days as a topless dancer are over." That brought down the house! Now I speak and whistle for churches, schools, and assorted gatherings, bringing the message that faith, laughter, and music helped me face breast cancer with a positive attitude.

***Patricia Derenburger**
Darlington, PA

Dear Cancer Club,

I have come to the conclusion that the Lord has a really weird sense of humor. Why else did he put all those organs and bits & pieces inside of us? So that doctors would have something to take out?

Before I'd even had my twelve surgeries, I tried to get my doctor to cooperate with me. But would he? No. So I taped a long, gray zipper to my tummy and insisted he come talk to me before he put me under. He did, and I whipped up my gown and said to please install this zipper. He was laughing so hard, he couldn't answer. The nurses on the floor were confused as to why my chart came to them with a zipper pinned to it. It took the doctor a while to come see me, as he'd come to the door, bust out laughing and walk away! So don't tell me I didn't try to simplify things for the medical profession. Keep the faith.

Shirley Timm
**** Wichita, KS***

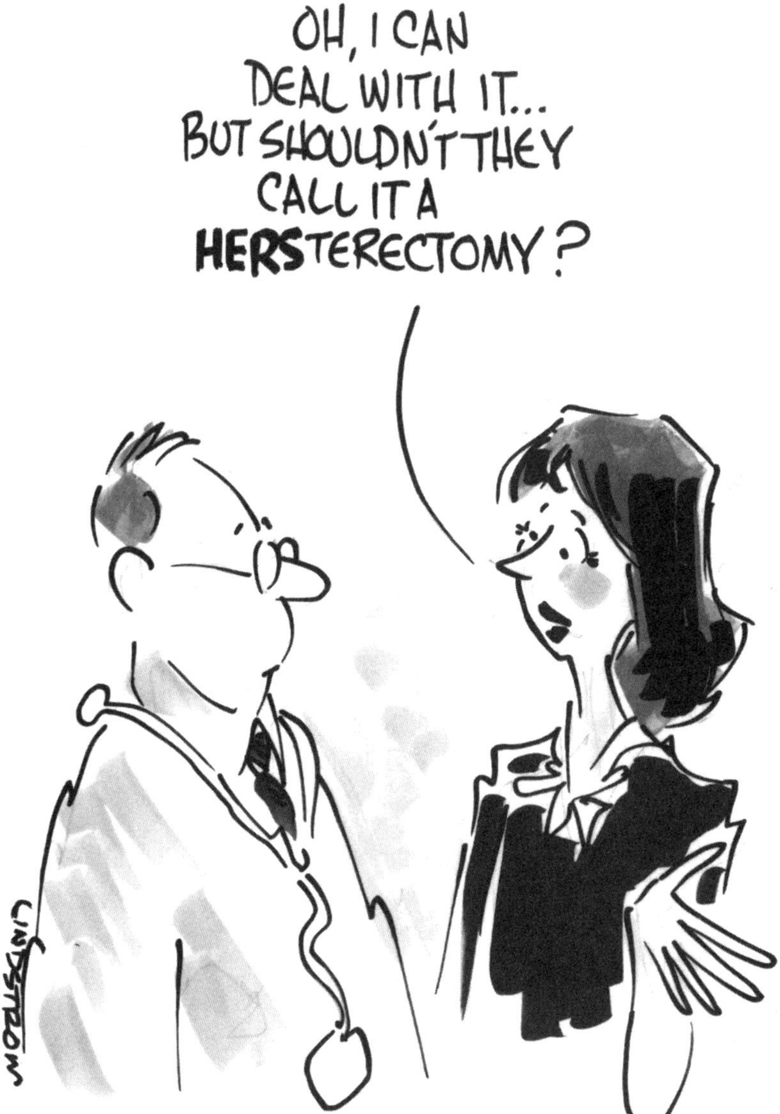
OH, I CAN DEAL WITH IT... BUT SHOULDN'T THEY CALL IT A HERSTERECTOMY?

Chapter 3
Laughter: It's a Family Affair

"A good laugh is sunshine in a house."

– William Thackeray

My boys were ten and eight when I was diagnosed with cancer. I made a bargain with my God that I wanted to live long enough to see them graduate from high school. When that had been accomplished, I went back to the bargaining table. Now it was seeing them both graduate from college.

Tim had me a bit worried there for a while. He dropped out of the Institute of Technology at the University of Minnesota after his junior year (it was already designated a five-year major) to go live in three Buddhist monasteries. But he got back on track (big sigh of relief), and both he and his younger brother Brooks graduated with flying colors and are gainfully employed. My bargain now? I want to see grandchildren. I may have to wait awhile …

Cancer never impacts just the patient. It impacts the entire family. And as I've traveled the world, meeting with hundreds of thousands of cancer patients and their families, the ones I see thriving and surviving are the families that can look back and laugh.

Vicki Woodyard, a writer who lives in Atlanta, Georgia and who has written jokes for Joan Rivers, Jay Leno, Jeff Foxworthy, and more, has this to say about incorporating humor into the family:

Two years ago, my husband Bob was diagnosed with multiple myeloma. Since there is no known cure, remission was our best and brightest hope. Stimulating the immune system is Job #1 and joy is the path to healing.

When our two children were small, I cranked out one-liners for people like Joan Rivers, Phyllis Diller, and other standup comedians. Most of them did not know that our youngest child, Laurie, was dying of a rare childhood cancer. I had started writing humor before she got sick, so I figured—why quit now? Now when I needed it the most. When her little bald head showed signs of hair "spriglets" growing back, I told her that I hoped it didn't grow back like Phyllis Diller's!

Children give us the gift of being in the moment, as does humor, and we laughed as heartily as we cried. She graced us with her presence for seven years and all too soon, she was gone.

When her father was diagnosed with multiple myeloma, it seemed like the end of the world for me and our handsome thirty-something-year-old son. He had already been through the cancer wars with his beloved sister, but he was just a child. This time around, he helped his father and me live every minute to the max.

We are trying to make this cancer experience a family thing. And it isn't all bad. The benefits of having cancer may seem paradoxical, but they nevertheless exist. The first one that comes to mind is the freedom to put yourself first every day. I used to let a ringing phone come before myself. No more. I used to indulge in negative, depressing thoughts. I try not to do that now. You see, life is too precious to be squandered in being unfaithful to yourself. You deserve all the good things in life, but you won't get them until you make room for them.

I never forget my humor roots. A couple of years ago, I was attending a seminar where they asked us to divide up into small groups and find out what we had in common. One woman asked if we all dyed our hair, but then she looked at me and said, "Never mind."

I said, "Now wait a minute! I do dye my hair." Everyone looked at me—the one woman in the group with silver hair. "I do dye my hair," I said. "I'm a natural blond. I just like to get it dyed gray!"

The laughter almost collapsed our little card table. You have to look on the funny side, even on the not-so-funny days. Cancer is the worst of times and the best of times. Worst for obvious reasons, but the best for some not so obvious ones.

Guilt trips aren't as fun anymore. Trips to the doctor can end with a dinner anywhere you choose. Sex may become as rare as hair, but both have a good chance of coming back. Friends become more dear, and so does your very own self. Every day is a discovery. Every night is opening night.

Give thanks for having the ability to laugh and grin and giggle again. It's no sin. Cancer has come bearing its gift, and you have embraced the experience. Never again will you live as mechanically as you did before cancer struck. You want to be present in your own life. And you will be.

* * * * *

I owe a great deal of my survivorship to my family: for the laughs and the tears, for the hugs and the kisses, for the chores that were done to bring me relief, and for the strength I found in those I call "family."

Here are some funny family stories from The Cancer Club:

Dear Cancer Club,

In 1990, I was diagnosed with non-Hodgkin's lymphoma. I had to close my medical practice temporarily while undergoing intensive chemotherapy. I felt compelled to capture on paper what it felt to me—a doctor—to become a patient. This urge gave me my first taste of serious writing.

I learned I can write anywhere: in noisy gyms, hotel rooms, airplanes, radiology reception areas, and hospital rooms. My ability to write in medical settings has brought me comfort, sometimes in the form of comic relief. In 1993, one nurse at Stanford University came into my hospital room to take my vital signs when my regular nurse was on lunch break. I was in a chair, dressed in comfortable clothing, working on my laptop computer, my IV pole camouflaged against the wall.

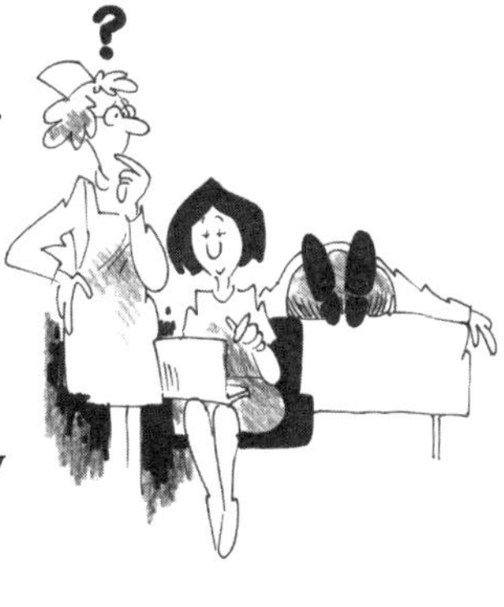

My husband, Ted, was taking a nap on the bed. She glanced at me, then looked at Ted.

"Uh, who's the patient here?"

** **Wendy S. Harpham, M.D.***
** **Dallas, TX***
* ***Author of*** **After Cancer. A Guide to Your New Life *and* When a Parent Has Cancer. A Guide to Caring for Your Children**

Dear Cancer Club,

A little laughter can go a long way. A lot can go even further.

My dad was trying to learn some of the household chores to help my mom, diagnosed with cancer. So he asked me to show him how to mop the kitchen floor. He was busy mopping the floor, while Mom and I chatted in the living room.

He stuck his head out the doorway and very seriously asks my mom, "Do you move the refrigerator when you do this?"

It was very funny. Unfortunately, my mom was having a "no hair day," and didn't quite see the humor in all this.

Poor guy. He really *is* trying. I hope my mom's sense of humor improves.

**** Susan Rosenquist***
**** Willows, CA***

* * * * *

Dear Cancer Club,

I often share a "wig story" about the look of horror on my two young teenage daughters' faces as we headed for a much-needed shopping spree after months of grueling chemo treatments for Hodgkin's.

On a great mother–daughter shopping mission, we entered the mall. Upon opening the door, a gust of wind blew the wig right off my head!

You should have seen their faces! All three of us stopped immediately in our tracks and held our breath as I quickly caught the wig, just as it was about to fly directly behind me.

As I promptly placed the wig back on my head, we started to giggle, then laughed while tears of sheer joy streamed down our faces.

Needless to say, the girls were extremely relieved and thankful that no one saw their bald mother at this tender time in their lives (ages 15 and 12). And so was I!

**** Francie Crawford***
**** New Hampton, IA***

Dear Cancer Club,

Prior to my chemotherapy treatment, Dr. Abrass told me and my husband that "They would be pumping me with the 'Super Plus' stuff," and that I'd lose every hair on my body.

The morning after my first treatment, my husband, Troy, leapt out of bed, frantically pacing, yelling, shaking his hands and his head, stating, "That medicine isn't working!" over and over again.

I was so sleepy and tired, I could hardly speak. He was so upset, he could barely tell me what the problem was. He just kept ranting and raving about, "Calling that doctor."

He actually thought my hair would be off, like when I raised my head from the pillow, there would be my hair!

This is the same man who told my surgeon to take my arms off if she needed to, when she informed us I'd need a mastectomy!

** Elaine McGraw Braman*
** Fernley, NV*

* * * * *

Dear Cancer Club,

While I convinced my oncologist to let me take my five-year-old daughter to Disneyland, I agreed to wear the mask on the airplane (so many germs!), and off we went. It was wonderful.

My husband was so much help and knew how tired I was. We had come home one night, and we were all eating take-out burgers, sitting on the bed (me with my hat off, and bald as a cue-ball).

I bit into my burger and my front tooth broke in half (chemo is hard on the teeth)! At least I didn't swallow it. But realizing what happened, I screamed (not really loud) and jumped up and looked in the mirror.

I turned around and looked at John and Emmy, and pointed to my mouth, the entire picture, and said, "Could I possibly get any uglier? Please, John, get me some Super Glue."

I was too exhausted and just went to sleep while my husband went in search of Polident (he really was the best). I spent the next few days with Polident and got my tooth fixed when we got home. It was pretty funny, and friends love to hear about it!

**** Andree Gordon***
**** Lebanon, NJ***

* * * * *

Dear Cancer Club,

On a Friday night, I attended a surprise reception for a friend who earned his doctorate at 75 years of age. We wore name tags to help him recall names and faces.

The next day, Saturday, I went to an open house for my second cousin's high school graduation. Upon leaving, a cousin came up to tell me he didn't think he could get used to calling me "Ronny."

I told him he didn't have to—he could continue calling me by my family nickname. When I left, I stepped in the restroom and noticed with horror: my name tag still on from the night before! I was the only relative guest with a name tag on it in all the pictures taken that afternoon! So much for "chemo brain!"

**** Ronalda Condiff***
**** St. Paul, MN***

* * * * *

Dear Cancer Club,

I do think that laughter is great therapy, but that chemotherapy wipes out my laughter for about a week. I'm writing this letter a week after chemo. So now I can start laughing again.

The other day, I needed to wash my scarves. Not realizing (because my body is fighting that "tired thing"), I put my wig in the washer along with all of my scarves, and washed everything. Wig and all …

I came to move the scarves to the dryer and noticed that my wig got washed also. I threw it on its side, and every single hair was sticking straight up. So then this morning, I went to put it on, and it was still sticking up, straight as a stick!

I went into the kitchen (where my husband was), and I told him that I was a dark-haired Phyllis Diller. He started to laugh!

Going back to the mirror, I noticed two white tags showing through the wig where my bangs used to be. I had the wig upside down! Talk about laughing! It was good for both of us to let some laughter come into our house.

** Carmen Branum*
** Oakdale, MN*

* * * * *

Dear Cancer Club,

I am a double cancer survivor: first colon, then breast, now eight years behind me.

I was visiting my daughter in Florida. While there, we were working in her yard: planting, digging up weeds, and so forth. I was wearing a camp shirt that buttoned down the front, and a "cool" bra with my prosthesis. I had worn it before without any problems. It doesn't have prosthesis pockets, but I do have pocket bras that I wear most of the time.

I was weeding around the stone walkway and came upon a weed that was connected to lots of off-shoots. I got a little too rambunctious, trying to pull the entire weed, when my prosthesis fell out on the sidewalk with a plop. I looked around and reached down, wiped my "boob" off very carefully and replaced it in the pocketless bra.

I heard the snickers, but very nonchalantly went about my weeding chore. My daughter just about lost it when she realized what I had just done! We had some good laughs about it later. We need good laughter and serious hugs during our recovery.

** Norma Jones*
** Rising Sun, MD*

Dear Cancer Club,

In July 2007, my husband Jim and I took a wonderful trip to Italy for two weeks. At that time, I had been breast-cancer-free for four years, having undergone a bilateral mastectomy with no reconstruction. Sometimes I wore prostheses in my bra, and other times I went braless.

When in Turin, we decided to walk to the train station a mile from our hotel just to see the variety of destinations offered. I had left my prostheses back at the room.

Suddenly, a sign caught our attention: "Train to Bra in 20 minutes." After a moment to reflect, I quipped, "Let's not go there." We both got a good chuckle as we sauntered back to the hotel, hand in hand, marveling at another funny moment in the life of this cancer survivor.

* ***Jan Hasak***
* ***Chico, CA***
* ***Author of* Mourning Has Broken: Reflections on Surviving Cancer**

* * * * *

Dear Cancer Club,

Here's one that might make you smile. My husband (diagnosed in February, 2004) decided there are some things he wants to do and not put off in his life—ride the Dragon's tail (motorcycle), get some more tattoos, etc. One recent thing: he's been getting some piercings. After 20+ years of marriage, this was a first.

Long story short, he got two piercings on his chest. Let's just say, "Ow." Anyhow, I asked him why that, and it was his answer that started my giggle. He said that he really dislikes his 12 inch scar on his stomach when he takes his shirt off, and the piercings give him something else to look at that he likes. Okay … here's the giggle.

When he takes his shirt off, he has two barbells (shuddering as I write this), a 12" scar in his stomach area, and drum roll please … a HERNIA between them both that sticks out and can't be repaired for at least another year. And to wrap this up, let's just say that he doesn't have the flattest stomach to begin with, and can't do crunches or lift weights because of the hernia. And, getting better, he never gets out in the sun.

Yeah, those piercings will distract them from noticing the scar. Oy! But, and this is a big but, it makes him feel good about himself, and that is what is important, I guess. Take care, and I try to laugh every day!

** Jill Collins*
** West Virginia*

* * * * *

Dear Cancer Club,

I want to update you on my health. I'm cancer free! I finished my chemo almost a year ago this past April, and my radiation treatment a year ago August. My radiation got delayed because I had an accident Memorial Day weekend and broke my right ankle.

After I finally got home from my daughter's house (I stayed there for about four weeks), I had a message on my answering machine from a gentleman I'd known for over 25 years. He wanted to know if he could come visit me, and thank me for the sympathy card I had sent him when his mother passed away. He visited for over two hours and asked if he could come back again.

Well, he kept coming back and he asked me to marry him. On September 5th, we'll celebrate our First Anniversary. He was a close friend of my late husband and they worked together for a time. I had been a widow for almost 21 years. I am very blessed to have him—and my good health!

** Elise Opper*
** Bowler, WI*

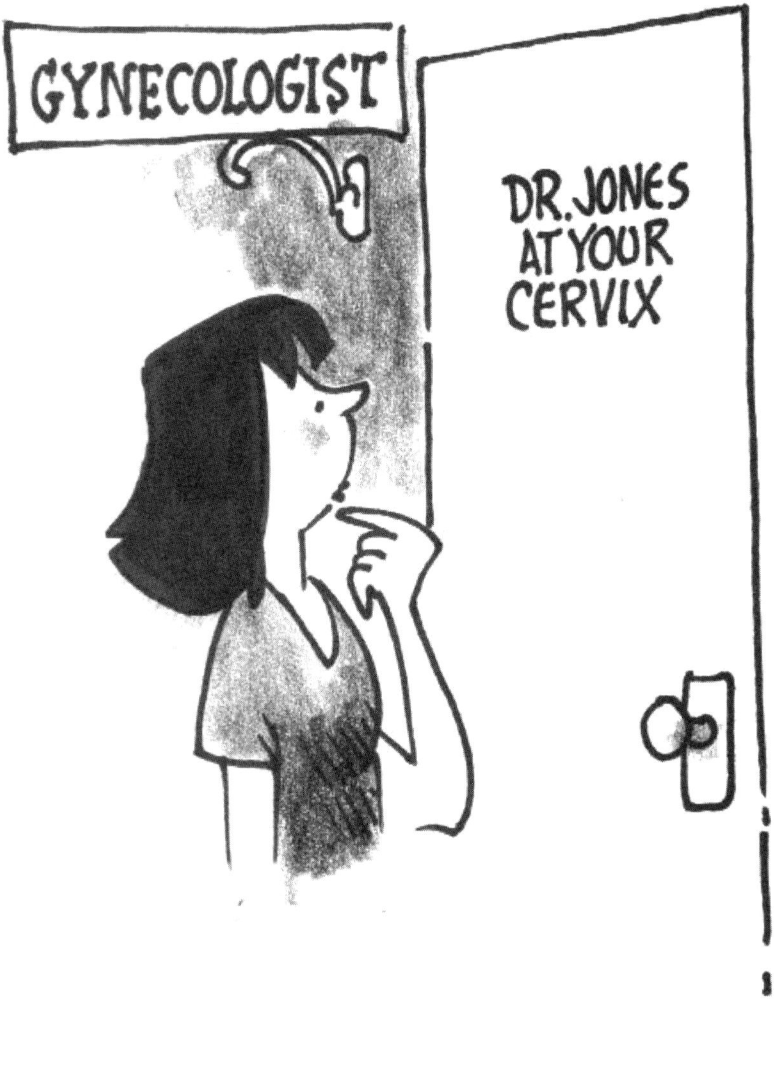
GYNECOLOGIST
DR. JONES
AT YOUR
CERVIX

Chapter 4: Kid's Comedy (Other Than Poop Jokes)

"From here to there, from there to here, funny things are everywhere!

– Dr. Seuss

I had only been home from the hospital following my cancer surgery for three days when Brooks asked me if he could have a friend over. Not wanting to disrupt *his* lifestyle, I said, "Sure, why not?"

The doorbell rang and there stood little David Vandermollen, the smallest child in the second grade. I only point this out because Brooks (now 24 and 6'3") was always the *largest* child in the second grade. I could never figure out how they had become such good friends. They looked like Mutt & Jeff.

But David stood there, and as I opened the door, he looked me in the eye and said, "Mrs. Clifford, I hear you have *CANCER*!" It's funny how kids never seem to have a problem saying that word! It reverberated throughout my entire household!

"Yes, I do, David."

"Did they get it all?" he asked me.

"Well, we certainly hope they did, David. And what they didn't get, we're going to get with some treatments over the next several months."

"Mrs. Clifford, I just want you to know that I said a prayer for you, and I hope you feel better."

Well … I had only been home for three days. My eyes welled up with tears, and I glanced behind me. My husband was standing in the kitchen door. He had tears rolling down his face. I squatted down to David's level, and said, "David, thank you so much for sharing that with me. That is so special!"

"No problem!" he said as he started bounding up the stairs.

Now in the meantime, Brooks had been listening to this entire conversation. And he had slowly been working his way down the stairs. So I stopped David, and I asked, "David, how did you know that I had cancer?" At which point, Brooks gave me one of those looks that only *your* child can give you. You know … the "*Duh, Mom*!" look!

"Mom," Brooks implored, "I shared it with my class during Show and Tell!!"

So much for privacy these days.

Stand-up comedian and professional entertainer Gavin Jerome and author of *Gavin Jerome's Comedy College How-to-Handbook*, shares his perspective on kids:

"Cancer Bites!"

Michael, a 68-pound warrior who was waging a battle with cancer, uttered that piece of wit and wisdom to me. Here I sit, on a picnic on an Iowa day in June that is so muggy, it feels like a rhino is sitting on my chest.

Every year Camp Sunnyside is engulfed with hundreds of kids who are dealing with the ravages of cancer. The Heart Connection is an organization dedicated to providing the camp experience for kids who are struggling with this dreaded disease. I was lucky enough to be able to provide a program for the kids, counselors, and staff.

But I have to be honest with you: I really didn't know what to expect. The one thing I didn't expect was in the air in abundance: Laughter. And lots of it.

Michael put it into perspective. "This is the one place where we get to be kids again." Another profound statement.

"So what are you going to do today?" I asked Michael.

"Everything," he said with a smile. "But first I'm going to make a friendship bracelet for that girl over there." He pointed to a sun-soaked girl wearing a canary yellow bandana. "That's Melanie. She's a babe."

I laughed for the first time since I sat down. Melanie was indeed something special. But after chemo took her hair, I'm guessing she didn't feel much like a babe. In Michael's eyes, however, she was. And soon that would be all that mattered. In a blink of an eye, Michael was off and running, but was quickly replaced by Rachael, a rambunctious redhead, all of seven years old.

Rachael sat in the front row of my presentation and laughed at everything I said. I wish all my audiences were full of Rachaels! "Here, I made this for you in the craft tent." She handed me an oversized piece of construction paper with a smiley face and the words, "THANKS FOR MAKING US LAFF," written in marshmallows and macaroni. "I would have written more, but I ate most of the marshmallows." I laughed again.

Rachael and I talked at length. We spoke of many things: of bumblebees and butterflies and Backstreet Boys. As Rachael rose to leave, I asked her one last question. "What's the best part of coming to this camp?" Rachael didn't hesitate. "Nobody here asks me any questions or thinks I look funny." And with those words still ringing in my ears, Rachael skipped away, probably in search of more marshmallows.

I sat there in silence and remembered a quote of Mark Twain's that I recently had read. He said, "The human race has only one effective weapon and that's laughter." Many of us forget that. These kids didn't. I sat there and watched these kids run, jump, and play and unleash the most powerful destructive force in their arsenal to repel the dragon they deal with on a daily basis. I sat there and watched as their laughter triumphantly declared, "YOU WILL NOT BEAT US, NOT TODAY. TODAY IS OUR DAY."

I glanced up and noticed Michael in the distance. He was talking to the sun-soaked girl wearing the canary yellow bandana. He whispered something in her ear. A friendship bracelet exchanged hands. She blushed. She laughed.

Michael's words echoed in my mind. "Cancer bites."

I sat and watched as these kids used laughter to bite it back.

And now out the mouths of babes ...

Dear Cancer Club,

One of our radio stations in Sydney pays people to tell their most embarrassing stories. This one netted the winner a well-deserved $5,000...

I was due later in the week for an appointment with my gynecologist. Early one morning, I received a call from the doctor's office to tell me that I had been rescheduled for that morning at 9:30 a.m.

I had just packed everyone off to work and school, and it was already 8:45 a.m. The trip to the doctor's office took about 35 minutes, so I didn't have time to spare.

As most women do, I like to take a little extra effort over hygiene when making such visits. But this morning, I wasn't going to have time to make the full effort. So I rushed upstairs, threw off my dressing gown, and wet the washcloth that was sitting next to the sink. I gave myself a quick wash in "that area" to make sure it was at least presentable.

I threw the washcloth in the clothes basket, donned some clothes, hopped in the car, and raced to my appointment. I was in the waiting room only a few minutes when I was called in.

Knowing the procedure, as I'm sure most women do, I hopped up on the table, looked over at the other side of the room, and pretended that I was in Paris or some other place a million miles away.

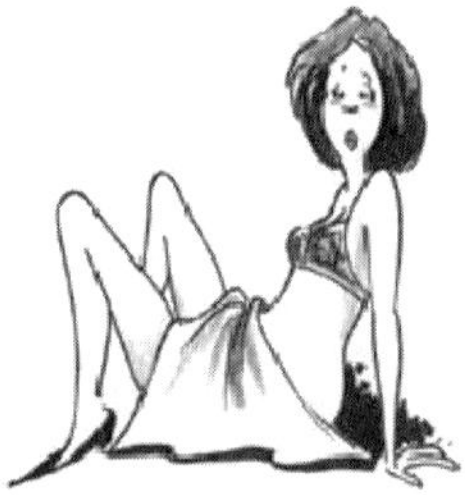

I was a little surprised when the doctor said, "*My*. We have made an extra effort this morning, haven't we?"

When the appointment was over, I heaved a sigh of relief and went home. The rest of the day was normal—some shopping, cleaning, cooking, etc.

After school when my six-year-old daughter was playing, she called out from the bathroom, "Mum, where's my washcloth?"

I told her to get another one from the cupboard.

She replied, "No, Mum. I need the one that was here by the sink. It had all my glitter and sparkles in it."

**** Keri Walsh***
**** Sydney, Australia***

*****

Dear Cancer Club,

I am a breast cancer survivor, and your humor is wonderful. Humor helped me get through my chemo and radiation, and all that came with it.

My son was in fifth grade at the time. When my hair had all fallen out, he told me, "Mom, I'll polish your head for a quarter!"

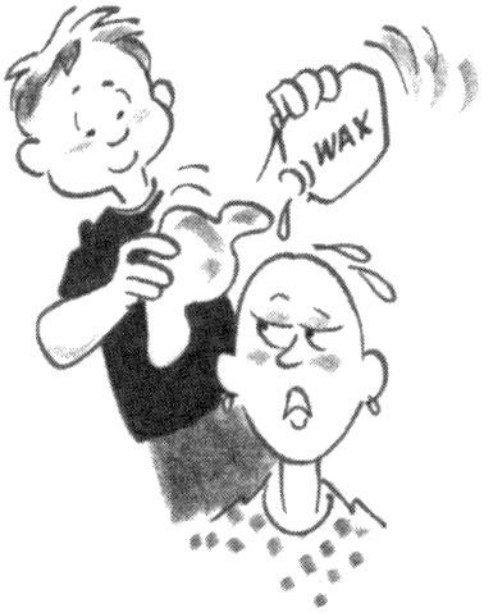

I was afraid to ask him what he was going to use to polish it! When he said that, I knew he was going to be okay with my "adventure."

**** Sharon Byars***
**** Killeen, TX***

*****

Dear Cancer Club,

Here is a poem written for me by my son, Corey. Enjoy!

Survivor

I remember the look on Mom's face
We knew something was wrong.
The diagnosis was Cancer. No, not my Mom!
So weeks of treatment lay ahead.
And with the first session of chemo, she lost the hair off her head!
Her long hair was gone, and that was tough.
For some thirty days, Mom had radiation every morning.

And after three surgeries, she was tired and weak
But there was a bright light at the end of the tunnel.
Support groups and family pulled my Mom through.
As the signs of Cancer slowly disappeared,
Tears of joy came because we know Mom was going to be OK.
The best part of all is at the Relay for Life.
You see all the survivors standing tall, United they Stand.
How proud I felt to see Mom walk those laps.
She's made it through the worst
Just headaches and hot flashes are all that's left.
One thing's for sure
My Mom's a Survivor, and don't forget that!

** Corey Birnstengel*
** Hastings, MN*

* * * * *

Dear Cancer Club,

I started chemo last month for breast cancer that has metastasized to my bones. I bought my first convertible a couple of years ago, so when the doctor told me that my hair would fall out in 20 to 21 days, I told my husband to plan for a drive when I gave the word.

I just lucked out that on day 17, the second day of picking hair out of the shower drain, we were at a first communion party that was winding down, and the sun decided to peek out. I gave my husband the nod from across the room that it was time to go.

We have a lovely drive from Alton to Grafton, Illinois called the "River Road." It's a 13 mile drive along the Mississippi River, with the river to the left and beautiful bluffs to the right. It was the perfect place to let my hair out. Now I hope my hair is being used in eagle's and squirrel's nests. By the time we returned home,

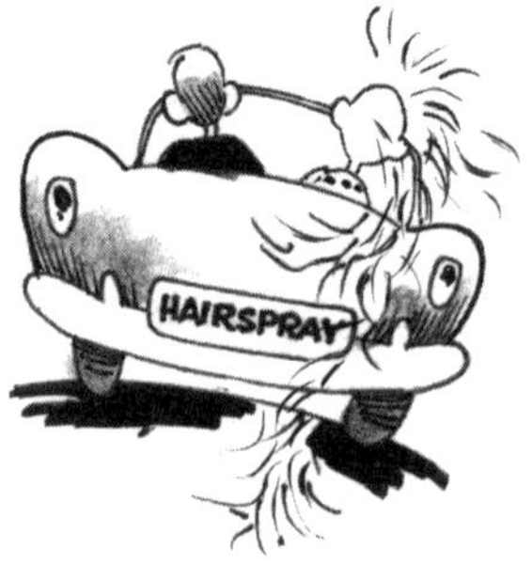

I told my kids that they were the only kids I knew who could say that *both* of their parents had comb-overs!

Feeling very self-conscious about my new baldness, I was wearing a hat and shopping for scarves at a department store. As I came around the corner of the accessories department, there was a little girl who looked like she was about three or four years old, shopping with her grandparents.

She looked up at and me and waved and smiled, and said, "Hi." I said, "Well, hi!"

And she said, "Well, don't you look pretty today!" It was obviously something that had been said to her before, but none-the-less, it made my day.

We should all take the time to enjoy the simple pleasures of everyday life, especially the words of a child, who apparently has great taste.

**** Rosemary Gaston***
**** Brighton, IL***

* * * * *

Dear Cancer Club,

I was telling my young daughter about my upcoming cancer surgery and treatments. I explained that I might become sick and lose my hair. My daughter turned to me and asked, "Mom, will it cure your stinky breath?"

**** Angie Olsen***
**** Kalispell, MT***

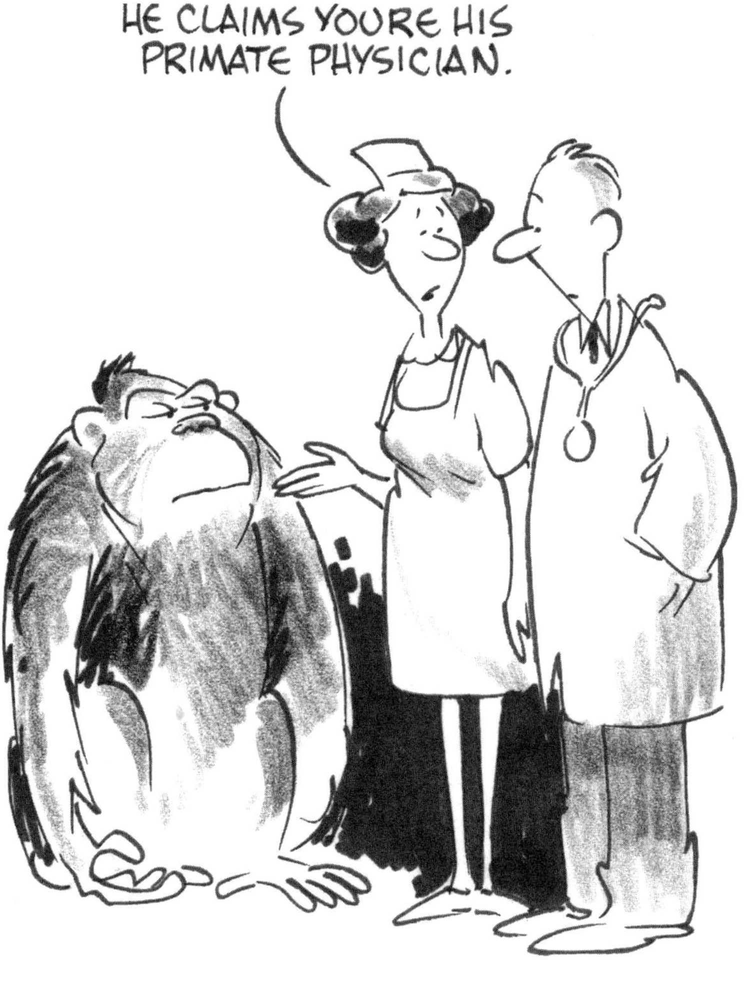
HE CLAIMS YOURE HIS PRIMATE PHYSICIAN.

Chapter 5:
Laughing with God

"Give me a sense of humor, Lord. Give me the grace to see a joke, to get some happiness from life, and pass it on to other folk."

– Chester Cathedral

The Pope died and went to the Pearly Gates. When he saw a long line to get in, he walked to the front to explain his rank, but his pleas fell on deaf ears.

"I'm the Pope," he boasted. "Are you telling me I have to go to the end of the line?"

"Sorry," said an Angel, "but we make no exceptions."

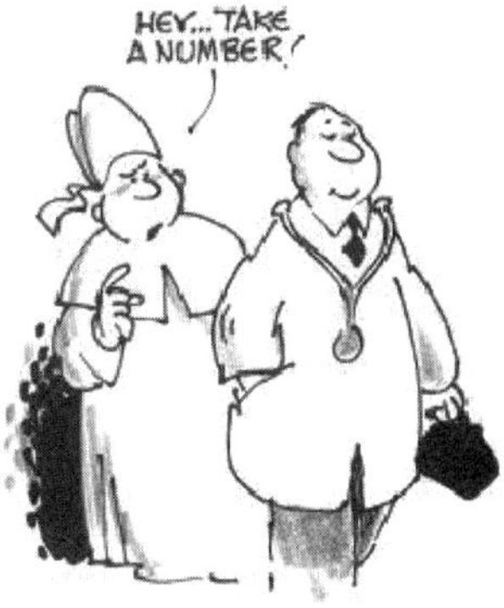

The Pope reluctantly went to the back of the line. A couple of hours passed, and he saw a young guy with a stethoscope walk to the head of the line. The Angel let him in.

The Pope was incensed. He stormed up to the Angel. "I thought you said there were no exceptions. But I saw you let that doctor in without waiting!"

With a glimmer in her eye, the Angel looked up. "That was no doctor," she said. "That was God. He just likes to pretend he's a doctor."

I know when I was diagnosed with cancer, my faith became even stronger. I knew that God had a plan for me, and that plan included The Cancer Club. Mark Darby is a speaker and author who specializes in helping people work well together. He has extensive training in theology and religion, and has been developing a spirituality of humor. He believes it is a gift from God:

Life is funny. We rush through life thinking that there will always be a tomorrow. Then someone says something like, "You have cancer" and suddenly, the tomorrows may be few in number. Developing a Humor Spirituality can not only help us find the humor in this situation, but can help us flourish during difficult times.

Spirituality has been defined as "The way we develop our relationship with God." Humor Spirituality develops our relationship with God using the wisdom of humor.

Humor Spirituality helps us to find meaning in the incongruities and paradoxes of life. The ultimate paradox is that we are all dying. Even though everyone's life span is limited, we spend all of our time denying the fact. A diagnosis of cancer can make us realize how precious life is, which is just how God sees life.

The Second Psalm tells us that "He who is throned in heaven laughs." God looks down at all our planning, scheduling, and mini-vanning and laughs. God laughs not at the people who, because of life-threatening illness, realize that life is limited; rather, God laughs at those who think life is a limitless credit card that will never have to be paid off.

The appropriate response to a diagnosis of cancer is laughter. You also cry, worry a great deal, and feel helpless. But you also laugh. If God, who sits in heaven caring for the entire universe laughs, who are we not to follow his example? God knew that you needed laughter to survive, thrive, and flourish.

In the book of Genesis, Sarah gives birth to a son at an old age. She exclaims, "God has given me cause to laugh and all who hear will laugh with me." So taken is she with God's gift of a son that she names the child Yetzach (Isaac), which means laughter. I think that this scripture teaches that in all hopeless situations, as Sarah found herself in, God will give birth to new possibilities which can only be celebrated with laughter.

Humor Spirituality teaches us to be on the lookout for these new possibilities, to recognize them as gifts from God, and to cherish them. These gifts can be very different for different people. For my aunt with uterine cancer, it was a day without nausea. Or it was one of those really strange hats you can wear when your hair falls out.

There is a parable told in the manner of the Ancient Doaist that gives us another final lesson on Humor Spirituality:

Mirth and Woe were walking on a beach when they saw a little child building a sand castle. Woe looked at the castle and said, "Needs some turrets."

Mirth looked at the castle and said, "How delightful."

Woe lived to be 80 years old, but it seemed longer. Mirth also lived to be 80 years old, but it did not seem long enough.

Humor Spirituality teaches us that it is not how long we live that makes our lives full, but how full we live that makes our life long.

* * * * *

Here's how some members of The Cancer Club found their Humor Spirituality …

Dear Cancer Club,

As I have faced my bouts with breast cancer, I have pictured myself as a dandelion wish: the tiny white wildflower that blooms each spring. Like the wish, cancer has taught me that life is fragile, and that life's journey is rarely predictable.

The wish usually is at the mercy of the wind and has no control over its direction. Cancer helped me to see how little control I have over my life. The wish must trust the wind and the elements, just as I trust my physicians and Creator.

A wish to me is synonymous with a hope or a dream. Every cancer patient must hold on to hope and dream of miracles.

***Vallee J. Kehoe**
***New Orleans, LA**

Dear Cancer Club,

Following is a poem I wrote. One afternoon, the words "came upon me."

Free

Once upon a time, you see
An awful breast disease got hold of me!
I cried and cried, and then I fought.
A cancer diagnosis I had not sought!
Today I'm healthy and wiser (I think)
And my world is quite rosy with shades of pink!
I still have doubt and an occasional fear
But God and His Angels are always near!

Sixteen years later, it is you I see
And still, hurrah, I am cancer free!
So on April 2nd, the birth date for me
No better present could there ever be!

***** Val Ohrt**
***** Sioux Falls, SD**

* * * * *

Dear Cancer Club,

Six months ago, I wrote and asked for healing prayers for my wife, Wendy Ripple. I am happy and blessed to write that following chemo and surgery, my wife and our family have been healed in a variety of ways.

I'm not sure how long you keep people on The Cancer Club Prayer List … but I do know how nice it is to hear the Good News that prayer works. Thank you for your ministry.

***** Michael Ripple**
***** St. Stephen's Episcopal Church*, **Fairview, PA**

Dear Cancer Club,

The Big "C"

The big "C" I heard someone call it.
Another just whispered the word.
That we don't even dare to say "cancer" out loud
Gives it power it doesn't deserve.

So I'm giving that letter new meaning
And refusing to give into fear
By reclaiming the power for you and for me
And by saying these words loud and clear:

Let the "C" be for "Cure" and "Compassion."
Let it stand for the "Candles" we light.
And a "Chorus" of voices shouting, "You 'Can'!"
To all who will take up this fight.

Let the "C" be for "Cash Contribution"
("Credit" or "Check" will work, too).
Let it stand for "Commitment" and "Checkups" and "Cheer,"
And the "Children" "Counting" on you.

Let it mean that we know our "Creator"
Is beside us each step of the way.
And remind us to "Call" on His strength and His love
And to "Celebrate" every new day.

To everyone facing this "Challenge,"
I say, "It's a fight we can win."
Tell all who will listen that, starting today,
The "C" is for "Courage," my friend.

****Kathy Cawthon***
****Hampton, VA***

Dear Cancer Club,

In 1987, my life fell apart! I was diagnosed with cancer; my boyfriend left me; and my business collapsed. However, I realized my life had to fall apart before it FELL together. I went into remission in 1988; my professional speaking career began to skyrocket in 1991; and in 1993 I decided I wanted to meet my soulmate!

The goal I set was to meet a wonderful man and get married. I listened and answered hundreds of ads and met about 74 men in two years. There was so much activity on my 800 line, the phone company asked if I wanted a block on it!

In 1994, I answered an ad that read, "Breathing, has pulse, and can eat without assistance. If you chuckled, please call."

We spoke, but never met. Approximately eight months later, I wrote a letter to God describing the type of man I wanted (I wrote in the present tense, and was very specific). The guy from the funny ad called. He had been cleaning his room and found my phone number behind his computer. We met and were engaged in three months. We married nine months later. Thank you, God, for listening.

** Marianna Nunes*
** Burlingame, CA*

Chapter 6: Finding Funny Friends

"Laughter is not at all a bad beginning to a friendship, and it is by far the best ending for one."

– Oscar Wilde

One of the best-loved humorists of the twentieth century, Bob Hope, lived to celebrate his 100th birthday. For some of us who have faced a diagnosis of cancer at a much younger age, living to 100 seems incomprehensible.

Hope got his first radio show back in 1938, and as his career continued to progress, he surrounded himself with the world's best comedy writers. Gene Perret, Hope's head writer from 1969 until Hope retired, said when Hope was traveling, he'd often run across a hot, local topic. He'd call and say, "Get me some gags about this." When Bob would call back a half hour later, he never said, "Hello," or "How are you?"

His first words were always, "Thrill me."

I think it's no coincidence that people who surround themselves with humor, such as Hope, live to be 100. "Thrill me" implies a life of looking for adventure—enjoying every moment; living in the here and now.

Another legendary humorist, George Burns, who also lived to a ripe old age of 100, used to say, "Laughter prevents hardening of the attitudes."

Living to 100 years old doesn't just happen. It takes hard work, faith, love, support, luck, and a strong sense of humor. But there is another extremely important ingredient: friendships. Next time you pick up the phone and call one of your best friends, instead of saying, "Hi, how are you?" why don't you try, "Thrill me." The responses you get may just set off enough laughter in your life to carry you to that 100-year mark.

Dr. Edward Dunkelblau (even he laughs when he pronounces his own name), an internationally known consultant and speaker on the topics of humor, health, and emotional intelligence, shared this with me about the importance of friends in the recovery process:

Ever since her mastectomy, Dolores was very depressed. She still went to work, but she rarely smiled and no longer would "shoot the bull" with her colleagues. However, one day, all of that changed. She was telling stories, laughing with her office mates and generally seemed brighter and more energetic.

Her good friend Anne noticed the difference and was curious about the change. She asked Dolores what was different. Dolores said, "Last Tuesday I just woke up, and I realized that my sense of humor was not in my left breast."

Where is your sense of humor located?

We all like to laugh, and have senses of humor. But sometimes our sense of humor becomes buried under the sadness and fear of a serious illness. Learning to laugh with disease is like switching on a nightlight in a dark, scary room.

We who are in the helping professions have found that humor and laughter have many therapeutic effects. Although there is conflicting research on whether a good laugh affects our ability to fight off illness, what we do know is that laughter feels good, lightens our mood, and enhances our creativity. It also helps us feel closer to one another and helps us to change our perspective. It makes hard tasks easier to tolerate and can shorten the most tedious of journeys. As Waleed Salameh says, "Life is full of pain and suffering. Humor allows us to realize that although there isn't much we can do about the pain of life, suffering is optional."

If you have cancer or know someone who does, I recommend that you do the following:

1.) *Recognize that we all have our very own timeline for being ready to laugh. Don't try to force or insist on humor.*
2.) *Be aware of your own anxiety about the illness. Sometimes feelings get expressed as laughter, when they are really something else like fear, hurt, or anger.*
3.) *Consider all kinds of humorous, playful supports and materials. Books, movies, puppets, DVDs, and props are a good start.*
4.) *Practice "no hurt" humor. Avoid sarcasm, sexist, racist, etc. jokes and humor. Humor can express empathy and closeness, but it can also distance us from others.*

5.) Let the people around you know when humor and laughter are appreciated.

Humor is all around us. It is low cost, has few side effects, and is not fattening. I encourage large doses on a daily basis.

* * * * *

What is it about sharing a good laugh with a friend that makes all of our pains and heartaches go away? I had one of the biggest laughs of my life with Cancer Club member Ronalda Condiff. Let me allow her to explain:

Dear Cancer Club,

I went to the book signing all properly dressed and eager to meet Christine. I arrived early and hung my jacket over my chair. Later I stood up to introduce myself to Christine and asked her for a picture of her with me for my cancer album. A co-worker took two pictures of us behind a bowl of marbles. I thanked Christine and went to my seat.

At some point, I noticed a different color black on my legs. Embarrassment set in. I had only my black "Cuddl Duds" leggings on! My "chemo brain" had not told me to put on my black slacks! I had my boots on and all, but no pants.

Needless to say, I did not move from the chair until I could put my jacket on to cover my rear. I did have Christine autograph my books, though. I do have my priorities!

Upon arriving home, I looked in the mirror to see my profile: jacket off, leggings cupped under my rear and falling in folds down my legs (not smooth like slacks!). What a humorous and unforgettable experience!

**** Ronalda Condiff***
**** St. Paul, MN***

* * * * *

Dear Cancer Club,

I have a wonderful friend, Tina, who accompanied me five out of six times to my chemotherapy treatments. (My husband, although very supportive in other ways, went with me the first time, but left the treatment room as soon as he saw the first needle!) Tina was my encourager, my strength, my prayer partner, and the one who kept me distracted as the chemo worked its way intravenously into my body. She would start up a new conversation if she noticed I was feeling shaky or restless.

Somewhere in the middle of my third treatment, I hit that uncomfortable phase, where I just wanted the plastic "bottles" over my head to be empty, so I could leave and go crash in my own bed. I had begun glancing up at them every few moments, just to find they were *still* half full.

Tina, noticing this, began a conversation. "I get to wondering sometimes just what God has in store for me for the rest of my life," she said. "I know it's got to be something good."

I ran some possibilities about the future of my own life quickly through my mind. I was hoping I might finally become an author—my life-long ambition. I had also been wondering if He might lead me sooner or later to somehow help other people going through similar experiences, such as I was presently going through.

Instead of dwelling on either of these, however, I was suddenly reminded of the few very blonde hair sprouts under my wig (where I had previously been a brunette), and a humorous thought came to mind. It came to my mind, but didn't make it to my mouth. I meant to say, "Maybe I will be a blonde model."

But because of the effect the chemo was having on my brain, what came out was, "Maybe I will be a blonde marble."

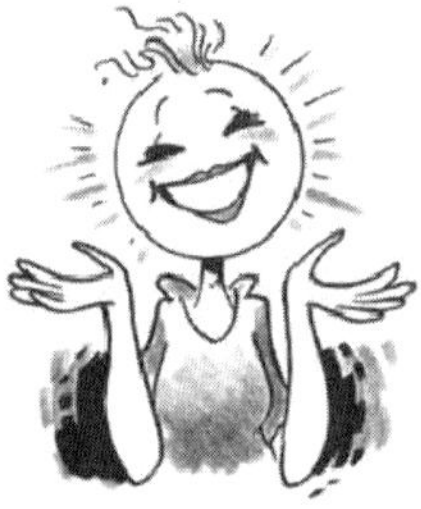

We both began laughing and laughing, and couldn't stop. The nurses didn't know what was wrong with us, and I was fearful that I might pull my IV needle loose! Needless to say, the rest of that treatment passed by quickly from that point on.

**** Susan Nunn***
**** Laurens, SC***

Dear Cancer Club,

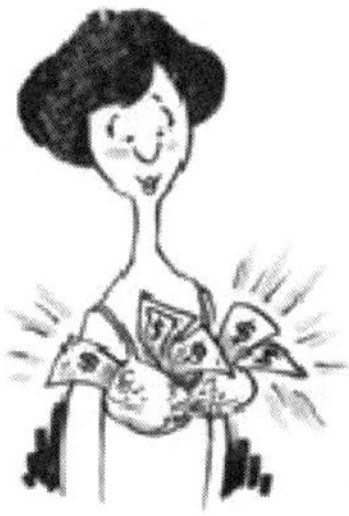

I am a recently diagnosed cancer patient and, like you, try to approach things with a positive attitude and a sense of humor. For example, every Friday I play cards with some friends. These are "high stakes" games: all of $2.00 per game. I told them early on that I needed money for my boob fund and got no sympathy whatsoever.

Then, the Friday before my surgery, they presented me with a gift. They said they were deeply concerned about me, so they took up a collection to provide me with a prosthesis: cotton balls! (I'm small busted, so it wouldn't take much).

Another friend gave me a note and a gift. The note said, "Since your top half will be out of commission for awhile, I thought your bottom half might like some attention." The gift was thong panties. Keep laughing!

* ***Rose A. Sodergren***
* ***Sun City, AZ***

* * * * *

Dear Cancer Club,

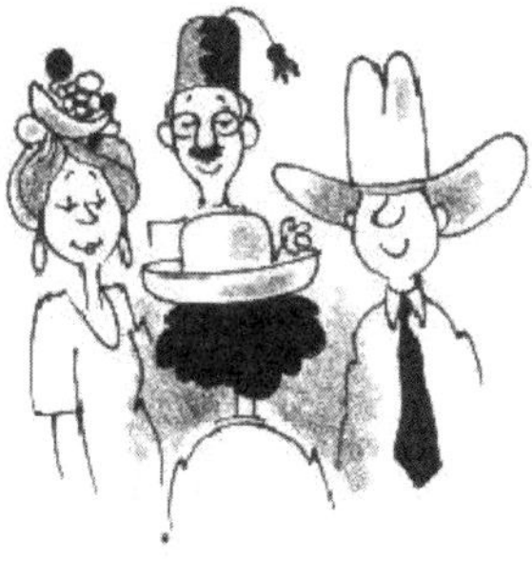

I have been recently diagnosed with non-Hodgkin's lymphoma and have just begun treatments. I'm a 47-year-old mother of three, and grandmother of three as well. I had told a few people at work that I would be wearing a hat to work last Friday. When I showed up, the entire building had on hats and were waiting for me in the hallway! It was great, and it made me feel so at ease. Twenty-five women—all in hats!

We had a great day with it, and now I know that I won't be uncomfortable in whatever I have to wear.

Thanks for a great way to handle this.

* ***Ashley Taylor***
* ***Meridian, MS***

Dear Cancer Club,

I was diagnosed with a particularly vicious kind of breast cancer in 1985. We were living in Montana in '85, but all our family was in Minnesota. Shortly after my mastectomy and before treatment started, we made a quick trip back to assure my worried relatives that I was still up and about. Our best friends were farmers, and had recently lost their entire farm in the flooding that had hit so many at that particular time.

My husband and I walked into Ken and Kay's kitchen, wondering just what we should say to them. It turned out that we shouldn't have worried because Ken convulsed us with his greeting.

"Well, Marlo, now you and I have something in common: we're both flat-busted!"

** Marlo Henneman*
** Ashby, MN*

* * * * *

Dear Cancer Club,

During my Mary Kay meetings, we often talk about clothing being "warm, cool, or neutral" in color. Once I tossed my wig (I went red) to my Director to demonstrate "warm." Everyone laughed. It's not everyone who can share their hair.

** Sue Erickson*
** Lake Orion, MI*

* * * * *

Dear Cancer Club,

Upon arrival at work the day before my scheduled double mastectomy/ reconstruction, my "work daughter" Jenny said to me, "You might notice something different about some employees today." Knowing that a majority of our healthcare employees are women, and not really noticing anything different at first, I said to her, "Are they going bra-less today?"

We giggled about that one until I was asked to go to the hospital's Christmas poinsettia tree in the lobby at noon. When I arrived, I was greeted by my many co-workers—who were all dressed in pink!

After hugs and tears, we posed for a photo in front of the poinsettia tree, which was a lovely shade of pink that year. I obviously was the only person NOT wearing pink that day, so the joke for the rest of the day was that I must not have received the memo!

** Francie Crawford*
** Mercy Medical Center, New Hampton, IA*

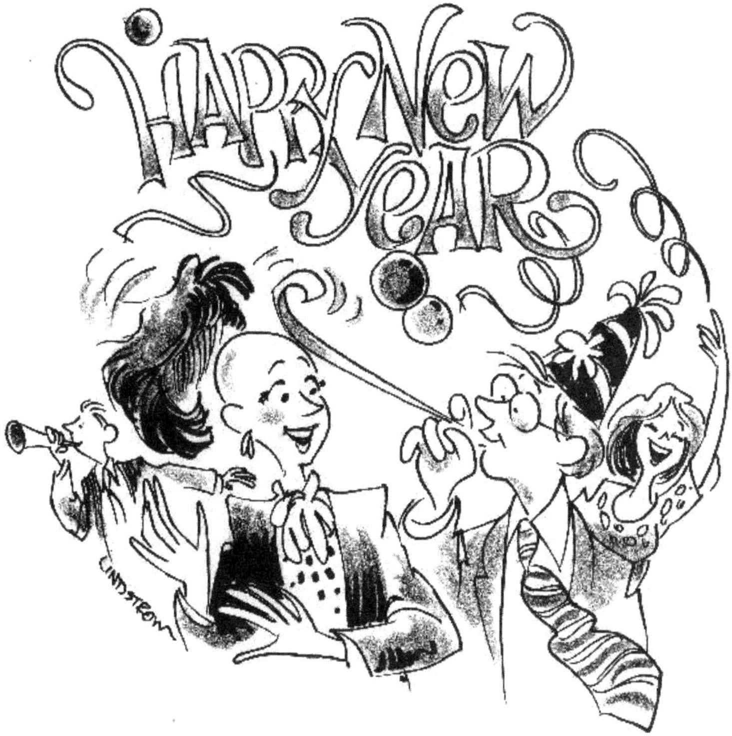
HAPPY NEW YEAR
LINDSTROM

Chapter 7
Funny You Asked ...

"They might not need me, but they might
I'll let my head be just in sight;
A smile as small as mine might be
Precisely their necessity."

– Emily Dickinson

I will never forget the gestures of love and support that were offered to me seventeen years ago when I was going through my treatments. From the home-made meals coordinated by a friend and delivered three times per week, to the family that came over and helped me wrap Christmas presents and address holiday cards, I couldn't have done it without them.

I was a fiercely independent woman who had always helped everyone else. But I realized that I didn't want to go through my cancer journey alone. I needed people in my life. And the best way to let them in was to allow them to help.

The offers to help were sincere and heartfelt. Helping is a way to show you care. And since friends and family often feel helpless watching a loved one go through treatments, allowing them to help you gives them a sense of purpose: a sense that while they can't take away the pain, they can be there to offer support.

And by the way, greeting cancer patients with, "Hey, you're looking well!" may not be all bad. According to a study in *Health Psychology*, researchers in New Jersey conducted in-depth interviews with 851 men and women over age 50. The subjects' appearance was rated from #1 (sick) to #5 (very healthy). The subjects then rated their own health from #1 (poor) to #5 (excellent). Ten years later, those who were assessed to appear sick or less healthy were three times likelier to have passed away than those rated healthy. So next time you see your friend or loved one going through treatments, tell them, "You're lookin' gooooood!"

Cancer survivor Izzy Gesell, author of *Cancer and the Healing Power of Play*, and Head Honcho of Wide Angle Humor believes humor is the universal human resource:

It is generally agreed that a good sense—and the good use—of humor is an important human resource. Not as clear is why this is true, or how one becomes more skilled at humor. Let's look at an area—interpersonal relationships—where you can easily benefit from an expanded sense of humor.

Humor among people works like a thermostat—controlling the climate within the environment. It is a key component of the ambiance that greets and surrounds everyone who enters your physical or personal space. Simply put, positive humor fosters a warm and inviting feeling. It relaxes people. Humor (or the lack of it) defines the emotional state of a relationship in the same way lighting sets the tone in a theater production where changing lights indicate a shift in mood. In the theater, the illumination fills the holes and occupies the spaces between characters, events, and the sets.

In relationships, emotions illuminate what people feel. It is a language by which people join and identify a common universe. They consciously and unconsciously make statements through humor about themselves, their relationships, and their families that they find difficult to say otherwise. Have you ever walked into a room where a group of people are laughing and as soon as they are aware of your presence, the laughter stops? These people were stating truths they did not want to share with you because you ____________________. Fill in the blank with "have cancer," "are a different gender," or are "not part of the team."

In many ways, humor is a coping mechanism. When truth is too scary or difficult to face, it enables people to detach themselves from potentially emotionally threatening situations. The TV show MASH was an example of how humor can create moments of sharing and community that offset feelings of isolation, termination, and helplessness. And Bill Cosby believes, "If you can laugh at anything, you can survive it."

The quickest and most effective way to become more proficient at the skill of humor is to lighten-up on yourself. This will positively affect both the climate and the flow of honest communication, another direct and helpful result of humor. That's why they say, "A lot of truth is said in jest." Begin to use subtle but evident forms of humor. Wear humorous ties, interesting accessories, or keep your high school graduation picture visible. The idea is to expose your sense of humor without having to have other people laugh. It is important to be able to laugh about yourself in a self-effacing (not self-derogatory) way. Self-effacing is non-threatening to others. It is humor about things you DO. Self-derogatory is about who you ARE. In this way, you acknowledge the reality of the situation, show that you recognize your humanness, reduce everyone's embarrassment, and put yourself back in control.

Finally, for both selfish and altruistic reasons, it is important to know what makes other people happy, so you can bring them joy while making them feel appreciated and respected. Pay attention to what makes your friends, family members, or co-workers laugh or smile. The more you feed them humor they like, the more positive the climate becomes. And since humor is a skill, the more you practice these techniques, the more proficient you become.

* * * * *

Here are The Cancer Club's dozen suggestions of things you can do that will give any cancer patient pause to smile and say, "Wow, they really care!"

How Can I Help?

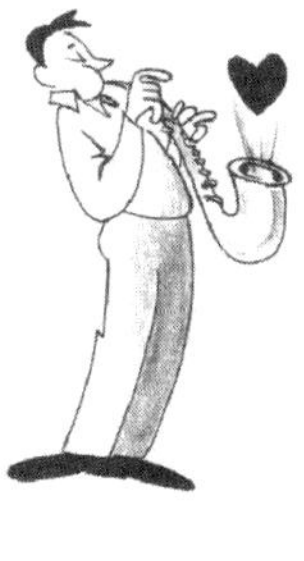

Music can truly soothe the soul. Make arrangements to have a musician come to the cancer patient's home or apartment for an hour. If the patient has a piano, hire a pianist. If not, a harpist, flutist, or even harmonica player can bring an hour of relaxation and joy to any cancer patient. Contact your local colleges, churches, or even high schools to see if you can find a volunteer. Then make arrangements to join your friend or loved one for your own special concert. It will be an hour you will never forget!

To Cancer Patients:

Sit back, relax and let the joy of music transpose you to another time and place. Allow your family member or friend to treat you to a special concert created especially for you. Have some hot chocolate, hot cider, or even a bottle of wine on hand to enjoy this special treat. You just might be tempted to take up lessons on an instrument of your own!

"May you have a song in your heart, a smile on your lips, and nothing but joy at your finger tips."

– An Irish Blessing

How Can I Help?

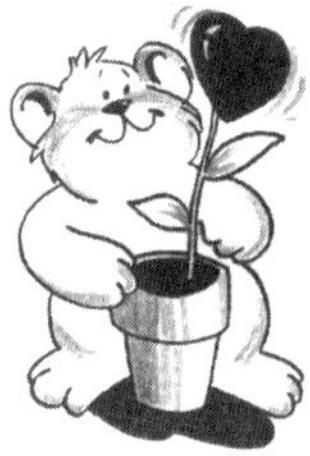

Start a collection of something whimsical or comforting that can help your friend or loved one diagnosed with cancer find something to focus on. If the patient is into pets, an array of stuffed, ceramic, glass, paper, or china bears, rabbits, cats, or pigs can become a friendly bedside support group. Marbles, quilts, or exquisite rocks for an outdoor rock garden can be given by all those who come to visit. Soon the patient will have an accumulation of items that will remind them daily how much people care for them.

To Cancer Patients:

If you have always wanted to start a collection or already have the beginnings of one, spread the word that you hope to have the world's best collection of tea cups, humor videos, or bird houses by the time you finish your treatments. Your friends and family will have a ball searching high and low for that very special "one," and it will give you something to concentrate on besides your treatments. Happy collecting!

"I realize that humor isn't for everyone. It's only for people who want to have fun, enjoy life, and feel alive."

– Anne Wilson Schaef

How Can I Help?

The healing power of writing or journaling has long been shown to boost the spirits of cancer patients. Next time you come by for a visit, bring a brightly colored journal or notepad to help your friend or loved one get started documenting their journey. A beautiful pen and pencil set along with an instamatic camera can be just the tools to help get that diary "off the ground." It may not seem funny right now to be losing your hair, for example, but months from now—when it's all grown back—you will both be able to look back and laugh.

To Cancer Patients:

It can be a stress reliever and "mind organizer" to write down your emotions, feelings, frustrations, and successes as you journey on the road to recovery. Get a "writing buddy" who can help you document your story and take pictures along the way. One day soon, it will all be behind you, and you'll be glad you took the time to record the events that led to your recovery. And years from now, your posterity will be glad you took the time to share your story with all of them.

"There are some things so serious, you have to laugh at them."

– Niels Henrik David Bohr,
Danish physicist/chemist

How Can I Help?

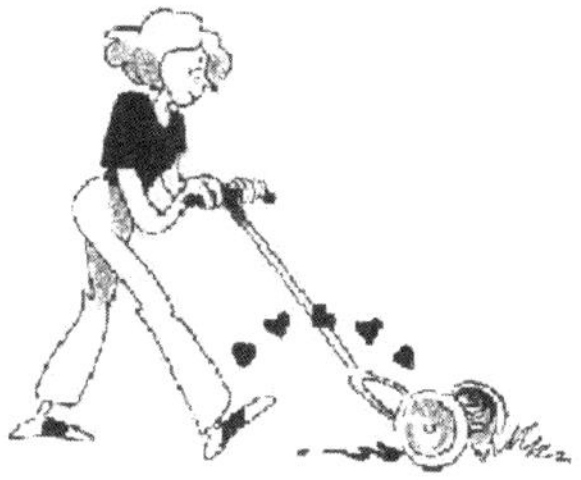

With the changing of the seasons comes a variety of outdoor tasks which can seem overwhelming to someone facing cancer. Offer to rake and bag leaves, trim trees and bushes, or plant bulbs to bring color to the yard in the spring. Washing windows or cleaning out gutters would be a fabulous way to help. Wash patio or porch furniture and cushions, or help put them away in the winter. Your friend or loved one will look around in delight when they know you've helped with the grounds clean-up!

To Cancer Patients:

When someone asks you, "What can I do to help?" take them up on their offer with a specific task around your yard or patio that will put your mind at ease. Pick a beautiful day to put your friends to work. They'll delight in the crisp autumn air, or the buds blossoming on the trees in spring. And the fact that they are also getting some good exercise never hurts! Then sit back, relax, and enjoy the season.

"A person without a sense of humor is like a wagon without springs—jolted by every pebble in the road."

– Henry Ward Beecher, American clergyman

How Can I Help?

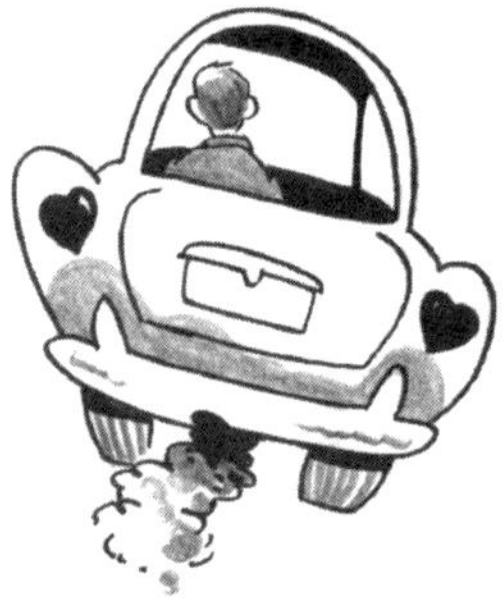

Let's face it … the only thing worse than having a diagnosis of cancer is car problems! But a mishap or breakdown—even routine maintenance—can be overwhelming to someone dealing with cancer. Offer to take the patient's car in for its routine check-up (oil change, fluid levels checked, tire pressure, etc.). Fill their car up with a tank of gas. Get the car washed and sprayed with a refreshing scent that will lift the patient's spirits. If an accident has occurred, offer to get an estimate, and schedule the appointment to get those dents removed. Your friend or loved one will be overwhelmed with your generous offer to help, and may just use the time you've saved them to take that necessary nap.

To Cancer Patients:

Hand over your car keys the next time someone asks you, "What can I do to help?" Relieve yourself of stressful activities such as check-ups for your vehicle when you have check-ups of your own to worry about. Let your friend/loved one know the location of your favorite gas station and/or body shop, and sit back and relax. After all, for today—someone else is doing the driving!

*"Our thoughts are like taxis; they take us where we want to go.
The way to get to happiness and health is to think happy, healthy thoughts."*

– V.E. Williams

How Can I Help?

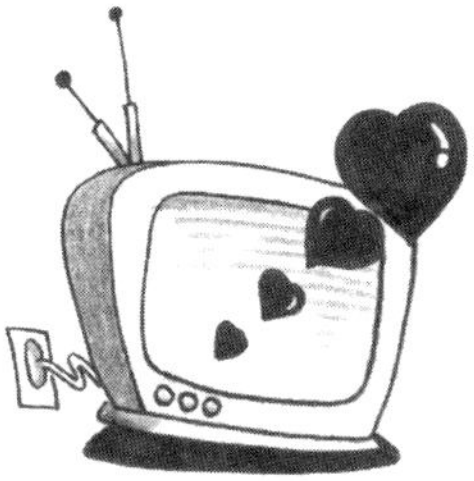

When friends and family members are far away from a loved one diagnosed with cancer, and travel is out of the question or nearly impossible, plan to make a DVD or CD of birthday greetings by sending a recording to share with the patient. Ask relatives and buddies to record words of encouragement along with wishes for the new year. Sharing funny memories and old stories in this way is a gift that will be enjoyed and remembered for many years to come.

To Cancer Patients:

Can't visit friends and family due to your treatments? No problem—just put your DVD in your player, wrap yourself up in a cozy blanket, and heat up some hot apple cider and popcorn. Enjoy messages and greetings from those you love who are with you in spirit, if not "in the flesh." And don't forget to laugh!

"Happiness lies first of all, in health."

– George William Curtis

How Can I Help?

We can probably remember the day we learned someone we love or care for has been diagnosed with cancer. The word "cancer" can spread through the telephone lines like wildfire, causing the cancer patient to feel like a fish in a fishbowl. During this critical time, use judgment as a family member or friend wisely, calling only the closest friends and family members of the patient, with their permission. Wait until you have accurate facts and information to share before making calls. Give the patient a few days to get acclimated to the news. The newly diagnosed patient is simply trying to overcome the shock of hearing those words, "I'm so sorry. You have cancer."

To Cancer Patients:

Call the person who is your closest companion and ask them to come over to comfort you. Share with them the news of your diagnosis, and allow yourself to cry and grieve. Then together, decide who else you need to call right away, and who should make the calls. Try to focus on just those people in your "inner circle," who you can trust and who will maintain your privacy.

"The two best physicians of them all—Dr. Laughter and Dr. Sleep."

– Dr. Gregory Dean, Jr.

How Can I Help?

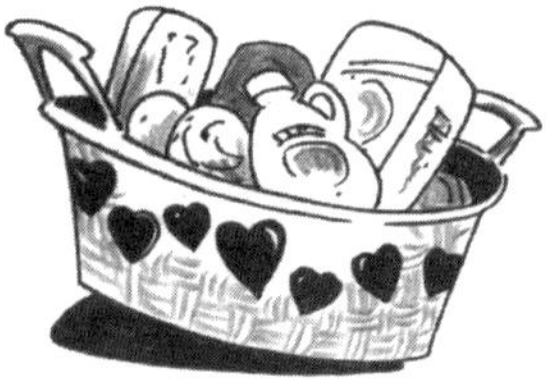

Are you looking for a whimsical or unusual way to help out a cancer patient? Buy an empty plastic laundry basket, and fill it with all kinds of treats. From household necessities such as laundry detergent, tissues, and soaps to bubble bath, shampoo, and a back scratcher. Mix and match all kinds of things that will bring joy and laughter to your friend or loved one. Or fill the basket to the brim with their favorite kind of candy or treat. Wrap a big bow around the basket and Ta Da! The perfect "Pick Me Up!"

To Cancer Patients:

Make a list of household items you need from the drug or grocery store, and let your friends do the shopping. When you have used all the things in your gift basket, forget about laundry! Use the basket to collect all the cards, notes and letters from well-wishers who are here to support you. You'll treasure these sentiments forever.

"The grand essentials of happiness are: something to do, something to love, and something to hope for ..."

– Allan K. Chalmers

How Can I Help?

With the start of a New Year, making resolutions for things in the past may seem just too overwhelming to a cancer patient. Instead, set aside time to come sit with your friend or loved one and design a "My Future" board. Write down the following categories:

family, friends/relationships, home, recreation/sports, job/business/career, financial and service/community/world.

Then, under each category, encourage your friend or loved one to think about where they would like to be in each of these categories five years from now. Looking ahead instead of looking behind is a great step on the road to positive thinking.

To Cancer Patients:

When we're diagnosed with cancer, it's easy to think and worry about the "here and now." Looking toward our future, and the things we still have left to accomplish and enjoy, is a terrific way to get our minds off the present. Have fun with your friend or loved one predicting the future. After all, we're here, and it's a great day to be alive!

"To be happy, drop the words 'if only' and substitute instead with 'next time'."

– Smiley Blanton, MD

How Can I Help?

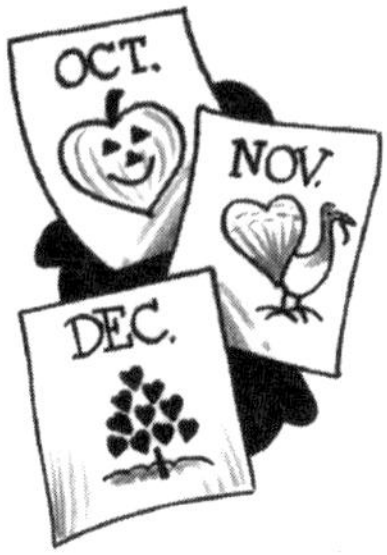

The last three months of the year are hectic for everyone—with or without a diagnosis of cancer. With Halloween and fall clean-up, Thanksgiving, and then the holidays, the mere thought of cooking, buying and wrapping presents, and decorating the home is enough to send any cancer patient back to bed. Offer to purchase Halloween candy, and bring over a pumpkin or two to set on the front porch. Bake a turkey with all the trimmings for Thanksgiving. Grab the holiday gift list and spend a day shopping for your friend or loved one's presents. Help put up or take down festive holiday decorations. It will surely be a load off the cancer patient's mind, and will help you get in the holiday spirit, too!

To Cancer Patients:

Don't be overwhelmed by the holidays just around the corner. Now is the time to ask people to help. Whether you need leaves raked, your walkway shoveled, or your car dug out of the snow, friends and family are just waiting to hear you say, "I could really use your help." Use this time to savor memories of holidays past, and remember: by this time next year, you'll really have something to celebrate!

"One of the best times to laugh and have fun is when you think you are too busy to do it"

– Dr. Chuck Ells

How Can I Help?

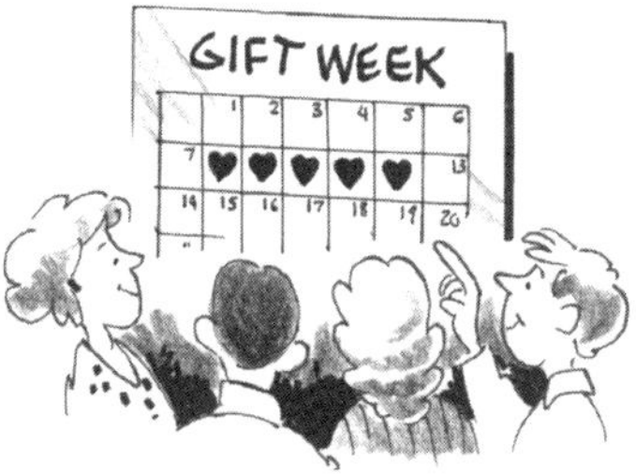

If you work with someone who has been diagnosed with cancer, offer to donate one of your vacation or sick days to the cancer patient to use as a day to recover from treatments. Go in together with several co-workers until you have a full week of vacation/sick days that can be offered to your friend. They will relish the time off work to catch up on sleep, recover from chemotherapy, or simply relax and enjoy a much-needed break. On the day off that you donate, send flowers to the cancer patient and a cheerful note wishing them a wonderful day.

To Cancer Patients:

If co-workers ask, "What can I do to help?" suggest the donation of a vacation day to help you improve your mental—as well as your physical—health. A day playing hooky may be just what the doctor prescribed!

"You cannot deal with the most serious things in the world unless you understand the most amusing."

– Winston Churchill

How Can I Help?

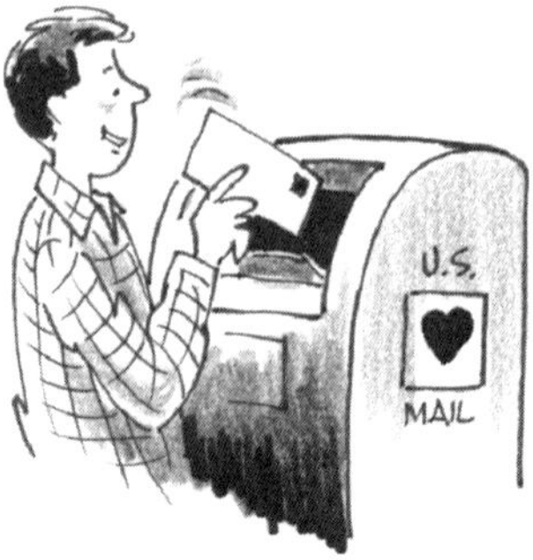

How often do we take the time, while people are here on earth, to tell them how much we care about them, and why we care about them so much? Take a few moments to write a letter to your friend or family member diagnosed with cancer that lets them know how special they are to you. Think of a fond memory, a shared gift of laughter, or a previous obstacle you overcame together, and write it down for them to remember. Remind the patient of their strong qualities (faith, spirit, strength, creativity), and encourage them to draw upon those qualities during this difficult time. You will brighten the patient's day with your gift of words, and they will always have your note or letter to remind them of your friendship.

To Cancer Patients:

Start a basket with all the gifts of notes and letters that are sent to you to lift your spirits. Keep the basket close at hand to read and reread when you are feeling down. Let the love and memories of your friends, family, neighbors, and co-workers fill you with joy as they share why they care for you so much. You'll treasure the basket of words forever, long after you've completed your treatments.

"Your living is determined not so much by what life brings to you as by the attitude you bring to life."

– John Miller

Chapter 8:
Fun with Food

"The sense of humor is like a pie in the face of adversity."

– Ruth Hamilton

Eating isn't always the most fun for people facing cancer treatments. Loss of taste, nausea, and other complications may inhibit patients from enjoying their meals and cleaning their plates. My suggestion is to find something that tastes good to you—graham crackers and banana bread were my things—and keep up your strength by eating whenever you can. Here are some fun ideas:

Dear Cancer Club,

I thought I'd share this great recipe with your readers:

POPPY SEED SLAW

Easy for the "non-cook"

One car in operating order　　　　Grocery with Deli

Get into car. Drive to nearest grocery store. Park car. Go into store and go directly to Deli Department. Take a number. When your number is called, ask for a small, medium, or large container of Poppy Seed Slaw. Don't forget to pay for the slaw on your way out of the store.

Preparation time depends on how far you live from the store.

YIELD: depends upon the size of container.

***** *Grace Katzenberger*
***** *St. Louis, MO*
***** *Note: Grace's recipe and hundreds more may be found in the Surviving Together with Family & Friends cookbook. 1-800-658-3241*

NOTE: Please consult with your doctor or oncologist before eating anything you may have questions about. Visit www.cancer.org for more details regarding specific foods.

GINGER POWER!

For thousands of years, ginger has been used to treat ailments ranging from the common cold to nausea and chronic pain. Scientists believe the active component gingerol is the power behind the plant's perks. While tests of how well it might relieve nausea and vomiting from chemotherapy are still ongoing, some people with cancer find that the taste or aroma of beverages and foods with ginger are soothing. Enjoy the flavor of fresh ginger in cookies, stir-fry, soups, or even tea. It's the real zing!

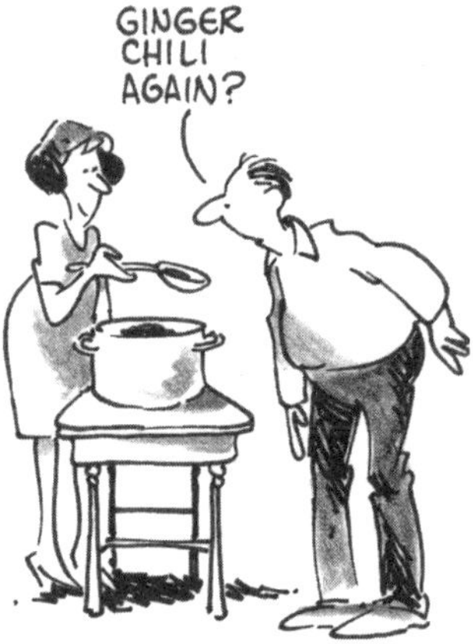

* * * * *

MARMALADE POWER!

Researchers at the University of Arizona were startled to find that eating orange and grapefruit peels (but not the juice or pulp) once a week or more cut the risk of squamous cell skin cancer by one-third. Their theory is that high concentrations of the antioxidant d-limonene in the oil of the peel migrates into the eater's skin. Next time you're hungry, peel away!

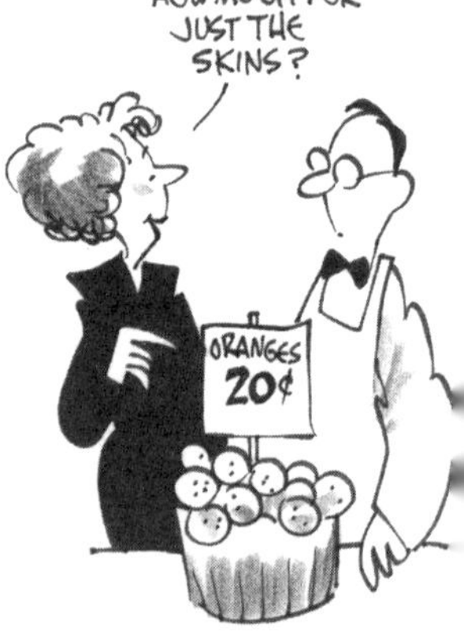

PEPPER POWER!

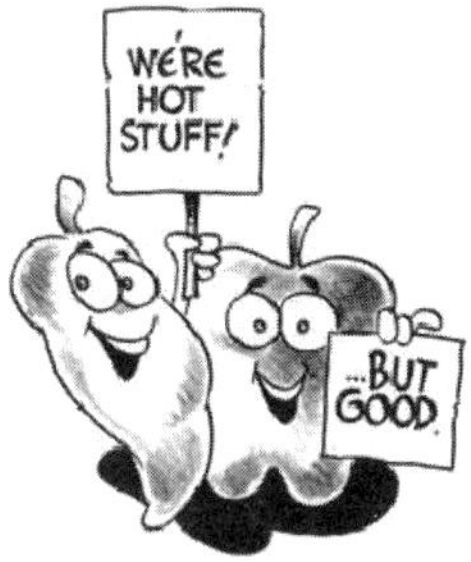

Looking for ways to spice up your food after chemo? Green and red chili peppers will not only add zip to your palate, but they may be somewhat useful for managing pain related to surgery and mouth sores due to chemotherapy and radiation therapy. The unique chemical Capsicum is the ingredient that gives peppers their fire and offers health benefits. They'll also clear up your sinus trouble!

* * * * *

BERRY POWER!

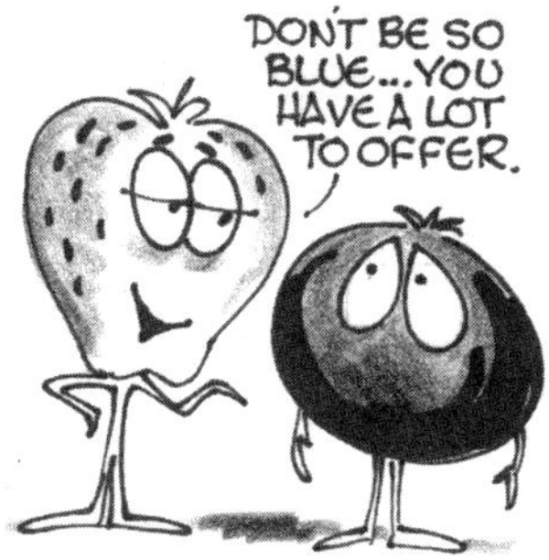

Blueberries, already known to contain potent antioxidants, have been found to be packed with yet another disease-fighting powerhouse: resveratrol. USDA chemist Agnes Rimando has found the berries brimming with this phytochemical, also found in grapes and wine. Antioxidants help mend the wear and tear of your cells, keeping them stronger and cancer-resistant. Lesser amounts of resveratrol have also been found in cranberries and huckleberries. Berry interesting ...

SUGAR POWER!

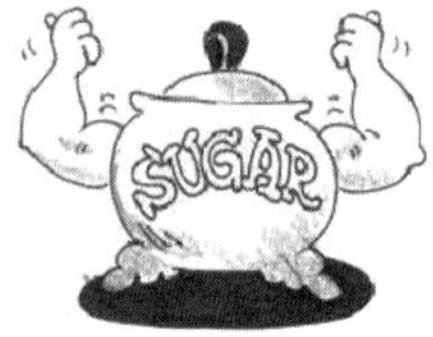

Wouldn't it be great to discover that all that sugar is actually *good* for you? Although glycoscience—the study of sugar's role in health—is still in its infancy, research shows that some sugars are just that. Glucose and galactose, the most common sugars, are not healthy. Sugar and sugar-sweetened drinks add large amounts of calories to the diet and may cause weight gain, which can affect cancer outcomes. However, other sugars found in corn, aloe vera and breast milk have been found to treat high cholesterol and obesity. So grab an orange and head to your treatments. Sweet, huh?

* * * * *

COFFEE POWER!

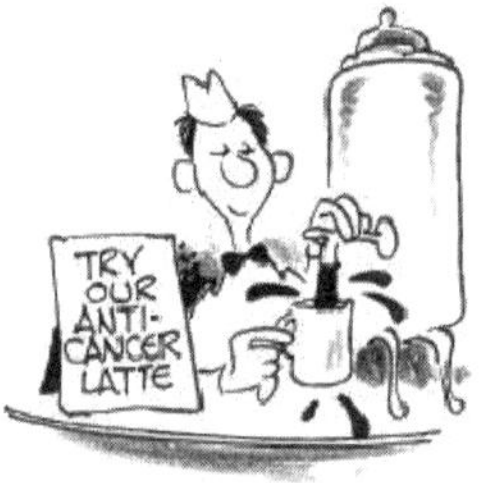

You may think it's what gets you going every morning, but inside every coffee bean are powerful antioxidants that may interrupt cancer cell growth. Dr. Thomas J. Slaga of the AMC Cancer Research Center in Denver developed a new way of roasting, which attributes almost as many antioxidants as a fruit or vegetable serving.

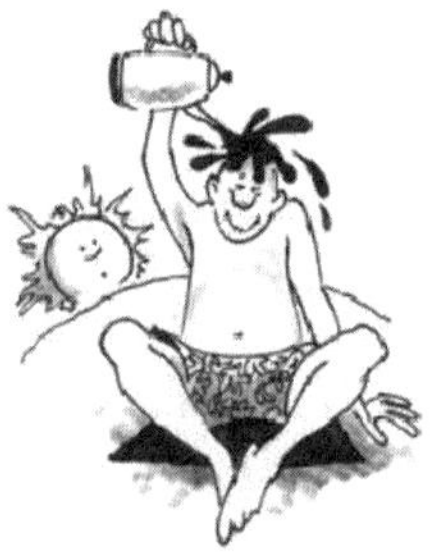

Think caffeine's only purpose is to keep you awake or start off your day? Rutgers University scientists believe topically applied caffeine may protect against sun-induced skin cancer. In a study using mice, one of three solutions was applied to their exposed skin. The solutions containing caffeine and a chemical in green tea called EGCG reduced benign tumors by 44% and malignant ones by 72%. Dr. Alan Coney stated, "Both ingredients may have increased the body's ability to destroy cells that contain damaged DNA." So next time you spill coffee on yourself, don't wipe it up … slather it on! It may save your life!

HERB POWER!

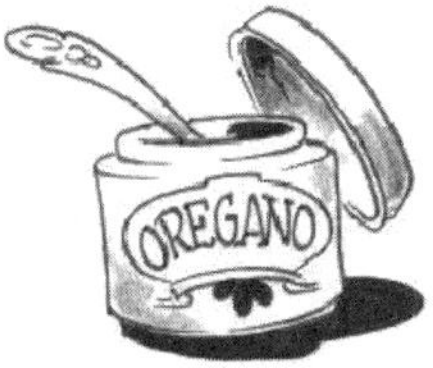

Researchers have found that herbs such as oregano, dill, thyme, and rosemary serve up stronger cancer protection than fruits and vegetables. It doesn't take a lot of seasoning—a single tablespoon of fresh oregano, for example, equals the antioxidant protection of an entire apple. So next time you sit down to enjoy your favorite Italian pasta, add a pinch of herbs and enjoy!

* * * * *

CHOCOLATE POWER!

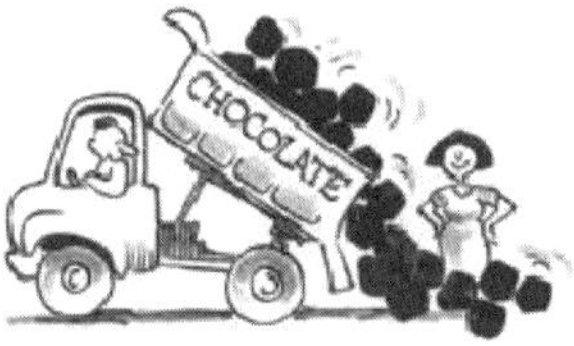

If you're anticipating feeling remorseful because of your increased chocolate consumption over Halloween, Easter, or the holidays, don't! Scientists at the American Chemical Society now believe chocolate may have some redeeming health features. Not only does chocolate contain high levels of antioxidants, which fight cancer, but it has high-quality antioxidants, which mean they work even better. So bite off those dark chocolate rabbit ears without feeling any guilt this year!

* * * * *

FIBER POWER!

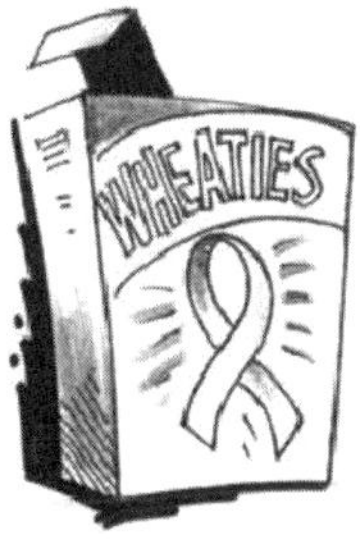

Wheaties aren't just for champions! Eating more cereal fiber—the kind found in whole-wheat bread, cereal, pasta, brown rice, and oats—may help you avoid one type of stomach cancer. Three Swedish studies found participants who consumed the most cereal fiber had a 70% lower risk of developing the cancer than those who consumed less. Cheerio!

TOMATO POWER!

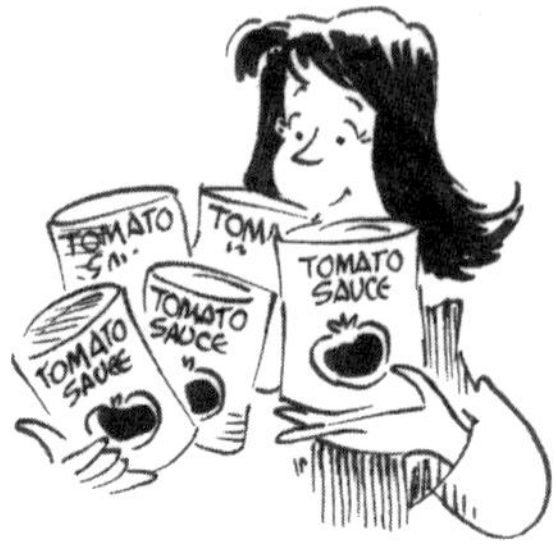

Ever since scientists announced that tomatoes could boost defenses against cancer, especially prostate, people have been consuming more tomatoes, tomato sauces, and tomato paste. Some, however, have been trying to cut corners by taking supplements containing lycopene, the ingredient that does the work. Ohio State University researchers have found that pills alone don't work, but tomatoes do. The study, which appeared in the *Journal of the National Cancer Institute,* believes that the little red tomato may contain several beneficial compounds. Pasta, anyone?

*****

KETCHUP POWER!

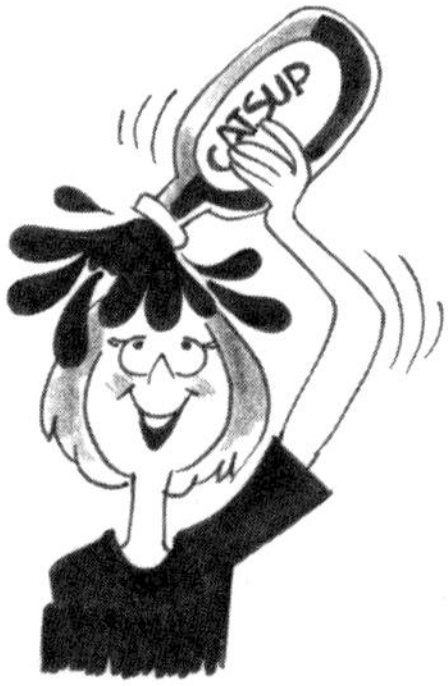

Live dangerously—glob on that ketchup! According to a study in the Journal of *The National Cancer Institute*, just two tablespoons of this sweet and salty condiment is better than a whole fresh tomato for getting lycopene, the powerful antioxidant that has been shown to lower the risk of lung, cervical, colon, and breast cancer. And no need to feel guilty: it's only 15 calories per tablespoon!

PEA POWER!

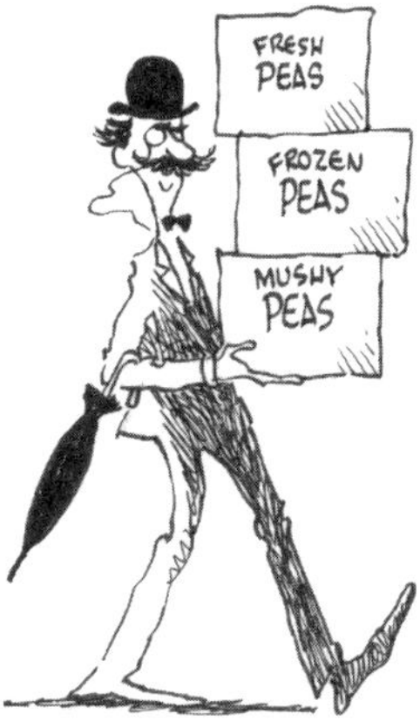

Researchers in Oxford, England discovered that men who ate green peas five times a week had a 65% lower risk of prostate cancer than men who ate peas less than three times a month. Their study compared 328 men with prostate cancer to a control group of 328 men. Besides passing the peas, please, other food items related to less prostate cancer: garlic, baked beans, and vitamin B6.

* * * * *

GARLIC POWER!

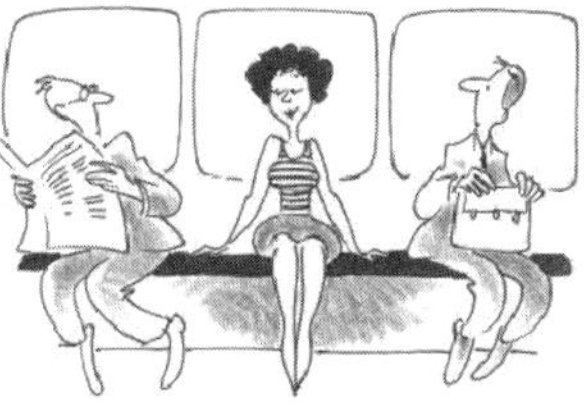

"A nickel will get you on the subway, but garlic will get you a seat." It may improve your longevity, said researchers in an Iowa Woman's Health Study. Women who ate garlic at least once a week showed a 32% lower risk of colon cancer. Garlic also appears to lower the risk of prostate cancer. If you and garlic don't get along, don't despair: onions, leeks, shallots, and chives offer several of the same cancer-fighting substances. Eat, repeat, and take that seat!

HONEY POWER!

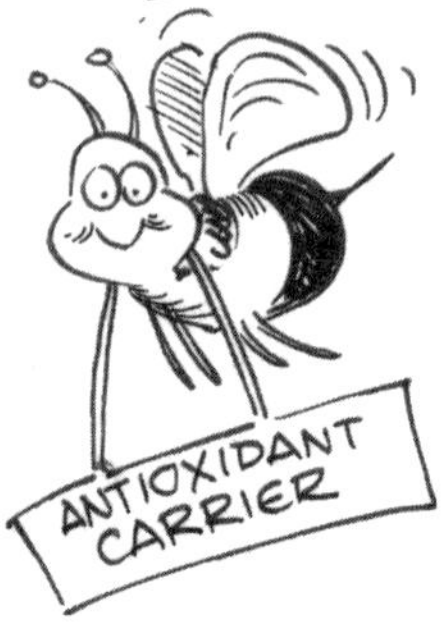

While honey has been used as a medicine for millennia, often rubbed on cuts and wounds to prevent bacteria growth, two studies suggest it may keep cancer from spreading as well. Turkish researchers applied an ointment of honey on instruments used to operate on cancerous tumors in mice, preventing secondary tumors that often grow along the instruments' path in such operations. Early studies hint that substances in the honey may help dissolve the cancer cells. Isn't that the bees' knees?

* * * * *

PIZZA POWER!

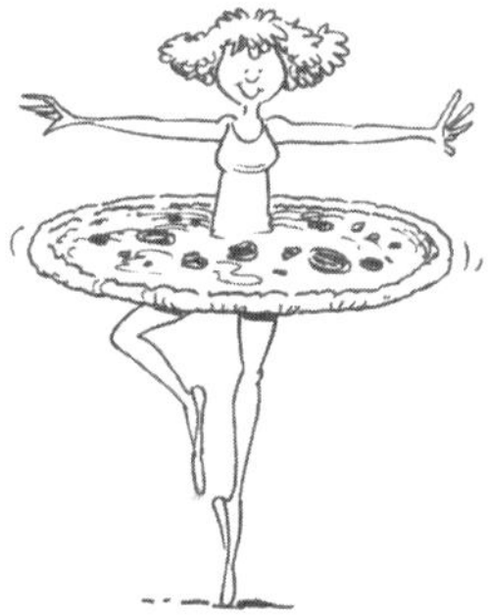

Proving pizza and spaghetti not only taste good, but are good for you, Clare M. Hasler, PhD, executive director of the University of Illinois Functional Foods for Health program in Chicago, reports that researchers found that women who ate the most tomatoes and other foods rich in the antioxidant lycopene were least likely to have precancerous changes on their pap smears. Lycopene, a carotenoid related to beta-carotene, gives red color to foods and is found not only in tomatoes, but watermelon, guava, papaya, and pink grapefruit. Bring on the sauce!

DAIRY POWER!

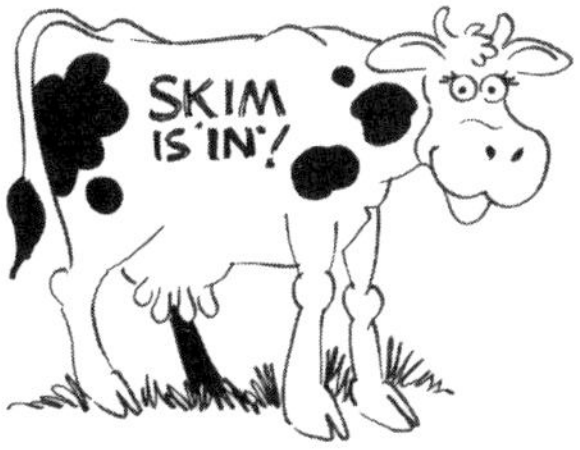

Greater consumption of low-fat milk, cheese, and yogurt appears to reduce the risk of developing colon cancer, according to Dr. Peter Holt, a professor of medicine at Columbia University. Published in the *Journal of The American Medical Association*, 70 patients with a history of colon polyps participated in the study. Half remained on a conventional diet while the rest increased their intake of low-fat dairy products. The group consuming more dairy products showed significant positive changes in colon cells, including reduction in the growth of abnormal cells.

* * * * *

WATER POWER!

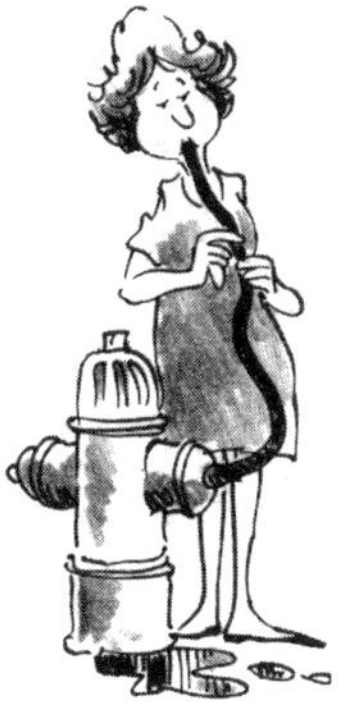

Researchers at the Fred Hutchinson Cancer Research Center in Seattle, WA concluded that women who drank more than four glasses of water a day had nearly half the odds of getting colon cancer as women who imbibed two glasses or less. Subjects who drank coffee, soda, or juice didn't budge their chances of trouble. Ann Shattuck, an epidemiologist, says water can turn your intestinal tract into an express train in which troublemakers have no chance to stop and loiter. A similar effect may keep cancer from taking hold in the urinary tract—home to your bladder, kidney, ureter, and others. So drink up and tap into H2O!!

APPLE POWER!

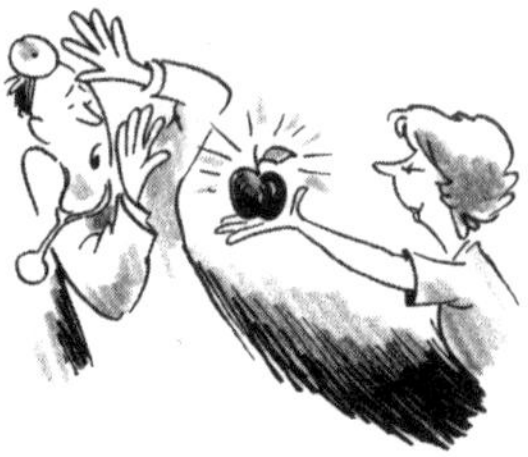

It's not just an old wives' tale: an apple a day DOES keep the doctor away! According to a University of Hawaii study, high apple consumption cuts the risk of lung cancer by 40% and as much as 60% in a Finnish study. Finns who consumed the most "flavonoids," a type of antioxidant concentrated in apples, were 20% less likely to develop cancer. Researchers suggest that such antioxidants inhibit enzymes that activate carcinogens. Antioxidants are more concentrated in the skin than the pulp, so remember: eat the whole thing!

Note: We can't think of a single bad thing about apples. Check for worms first.

Chapter 9: And Now for Some Really Silly Stuff

"A smile is a powerful weapon; you can even break ice with it."

– Author Unknown

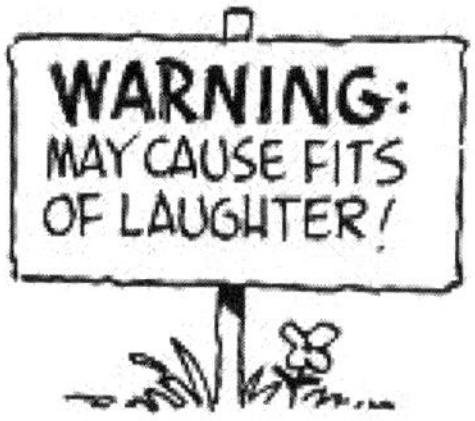

I used to rue the day when the computer was invented. My mailbox would fill up with hundreds of messages, most of them spam. But one thing did catch my attention: the thousands of jokes, anecdotes, and just plain facts people sent me that were humorous.

In this chapter, we will sit back, relax, and hopefully find a good laugh or two. But not without hearing first from Ann Weeks, DNS, RN and author of the weekly eNewsletter, *WEEKS OF FUN*:

Jest, Rest and Be Your Best!

Every year, a surprisingly large number of people—ill with serious illnesses, especially cancer—fool everyone and continue to live full and satisfying lives. When asked to what they attribute their "beating the odds," one and all respond, "A positive attitude with lots of humor and laughter."

Humor, and the laughter it brings, has many physical benefits, such as pain relief and a strengthened immune system. The psychological benefits are just as healing, and sometimes more immediate. Humor and laughter often relieve tension, increase our creativity, give us a sense of confidence and well-being, and help us put the situation into perspective. A sense of humor, after all, is our ability to appreciate the absurd in a situation.

Steve Allen, Jr., a physician and lecturer on humor and healing says, "Laughing is the signal that you can dance into the eye of a hurricane."

Julie Kurnitz, a New York actress, suffers from a rare chronic illness, Marfan Syndrome, which affects the connective tissue. She tells of an incident years ago while in London. She had a severe pain and knew that a major blood vessel had begun to tear due to her illness. She was very frightened as a taxi rushed her to the nearest hospital. She knew without immediate intervention, she would die.

Upon arriving at the hospital, the clerk said, "I'm terribly sorry, but we don't take emergency cases here," and handed her a walking map to the nearest hospital that did. Julie describes the map as having "little footprints like Arthur Murray used to show how to do the rumba. And then at the bottom of the map, it said, 'This map not to scale.' Even then, I knew that someday, this would be funny."

It has been my experience that many people cope with fear, disappointment, embarrassment, pain, and uncertainty with humor and laughter. We are better for it when we can laugh.

Humor also helps us look at life differently than we did just a few moments before. Often humor "peels" back the dull reality to reveal an ironic truth or an exaggeration.

* * * * *

Ann's words ring true as we examine some of the things that found our mailbox …

What If it's a Bad Joke?

In a study in the *Journal of The American Medical Association*, primary care doctors who take more time with their patients, encourage people to talk and inject a little humor are less likely to be sued for malpractice than doctors who rush their patients through.

R.I.P.

An elderly couple was lying in bed one morning, having just awakened from a good night's sleep. The husband took his wife's hand, and she responded, "Don't touch me."

"Why not," he asks.

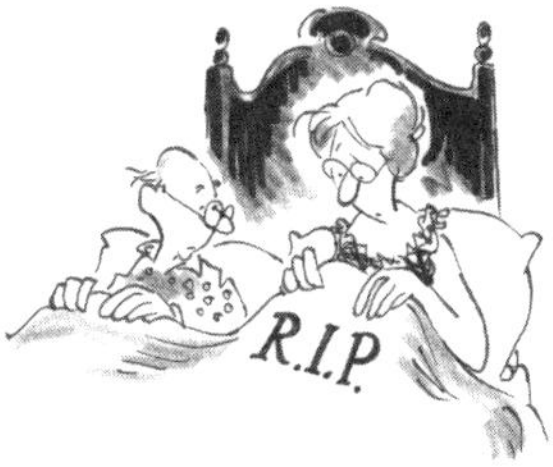

She answers back, "Because I'm dead."

The husband says to her, "What are you talking about? We're both lying here in bed together, talking to one another."

The wife says, "No, I'm definitely dead."

Her husband insists, "You're *not* dead. What in the world makes you think you're dead?"

His wife answered, "I know I'm dead because I woke up this morning, and nothing hurts!"

* * * * *

A distraught patient phoned her doctor's office. "Is it true," the woman wanted to know, "that the medication you prescribed has to be taken for the rest of my life?"

"Yes, I'm afraid so," the doctor told her.

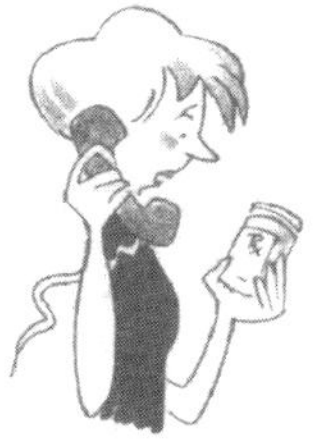

There was a moment of silence before the woman continued. "I'm wondering then, just how serious is my condition? This prescription is marked "NO REFILLS!"

(www.funnypart.com)

What's it Like to Be a Cancer Patient?

A woman was asked by a co-worker, "What's it like to be a cancer patient?"

The co-worker replied, "It is like being a pumpkin. God picks you from the patch, brings you in, and washes all the dirt off of you. Then He cuts off the top and scoops out all the yucky stuff. He removes the seeds of doubt, hate, murmuring, grumbling, faultfinding, greed, fear, etc. and then He carves you a new smiling face and puts His light inside of you to shine for all the world to see."

*****

On board a flight to Hawaii, the pilot announced, "That thump you heard was our last engine conking out. I'm really sorry to tell you this, but we are going to crash into the ocean."

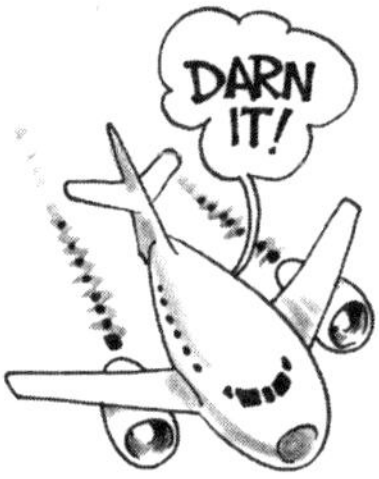

In the stunned silence that followed, an angry voice spoke out. "Darn it! That stupid doctor of mine! He said I was going to die of cancer. He lied!"

(www.support4change.com)

*****

Three sisters ages 92, 94 and 96 live in a house together. One night, the 96-year-old draws a bath. She puts her foot in and pauses. She yells to the other sisters, "Was I getting in or out of the bath?"

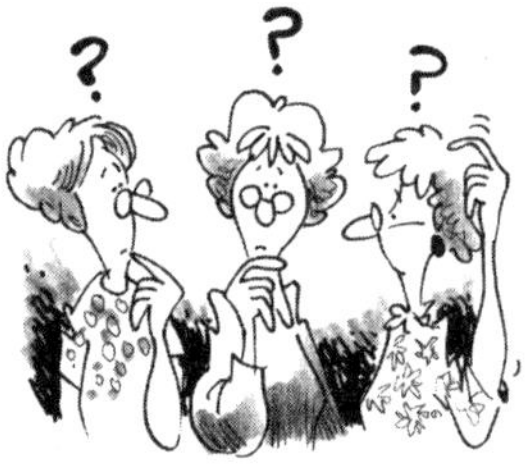

The 94-year-old yells back, "I don't know. I'll come up and see." She starts up the stairs and pauses. "Was I going up the stairs or down?"

The 92-year-old is sitting at the kitchen table having tea, listening to her sisters. She shakes her head and says, "I sure hope I never get that forgetful." She knocks on wood for good measure.

She then yells, "I'll come up and help both of you as soon as I see who's at the door."

As If Cancer Wasn't Enough!

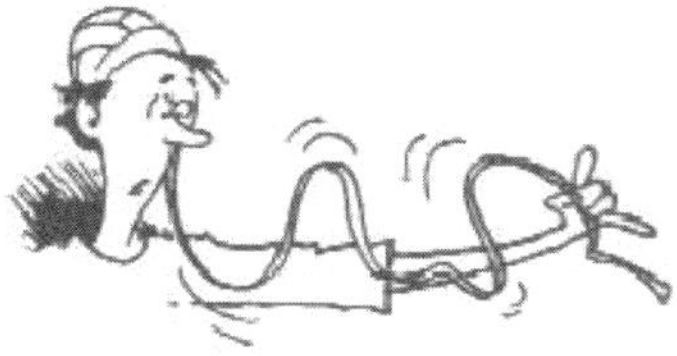

Goeran Rudolfsson, recovering from brain-tumor surgery in a hospital in Stockholm, Sweden, had been complaining about nasal congestion when he blew his nose and felt a non-natural substance flapping inside his nostril. When he stopped his gentle tugging, he was holding a 31" long cloth, apparently left inside accidently during his operation!

(www.miaminewtimes.com)

*****

Anyone Seen My Toothbrush?

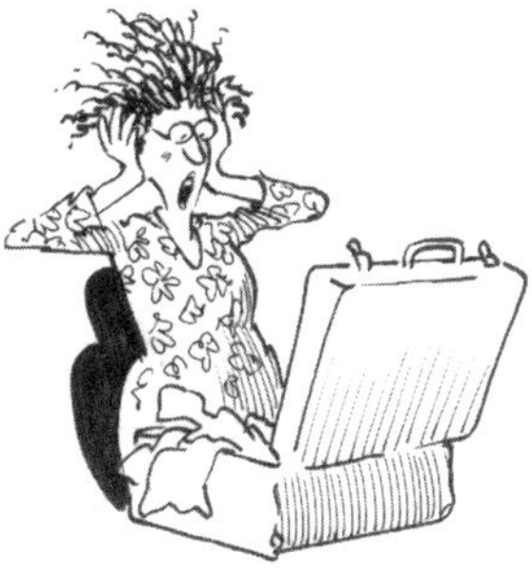

Virginia Broache returned home from the Bons Secours St. Mary's Hospital in Richmond, VA after having her cancerous bladder removed. Her nurse was unpacking for her and discovered among the "personal effects" the hospital had sent home with her was the actual bag with the just removed bladder. Said a hospital member, "We apologize."

(*News of the Weird*, ©Chuck Shepherd)

Who Burned My Lasagna?

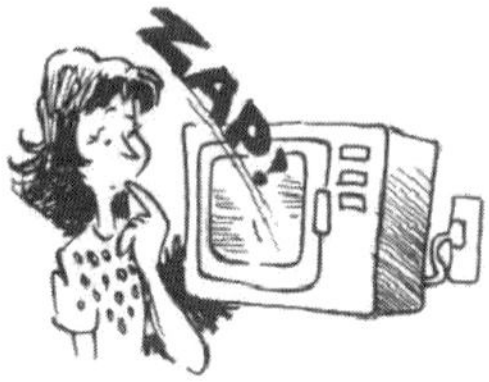

At the Presbyterian Hospital in Albuquerque, New Mexico, Anthony Valencia and Fitzgerald Vendever, both age 20, were arrested and accused of roaming the Intensive Care Unit, looking to steal patients' food off warming carts. A hospital spokeswoman was quoted as saying, "Actually, we've got some pretty good food down there."

*****

Forget About It!

A doctor tells a patient, "I have bad news and I have worse news."

"What's the bad news?"

"You have cancer," the doctor says.

The patient sinks. "What's the worse news?"

"You have Alzheimer's, too."

"Oh, well, that's good," says the relieved patient. "At least I don't have cancer."

(© Jimmy California, Maxim.com)

*****

Can I Get Some Aspirin With That Prescription?

Cooney hadn't been feeling well, but hated the thought of going to the doctor. Frieda finally talked him in to getting a physical by agreeing to get one herself.

After they had both been checked over, the doctor called Frieda aside and said, "I'm afraid Cooney has a very serious illness. In fact, it might be fatal. There are two things you can do to save his life. First, you'll have to fix him three home-cooked meals a day for the rest of his life. And second, you'll have to make love to him every day without fail."

Frieda pondered a moment and announced, "I'll break the news to Cooney."

So she stepped across the waiting room where he was sitting and announced, "Guess what, Cooney? You're gonna die."

*****

An Illinois man left the snow-filled streets of Chicago for a vacation in Florida. His wife was on a business trip and was planning to meet him there the next day.

When he reached his hotel in Florida, he decided to send his wife a quick e-mail. Unable to find the scrap of paper with her e-mail address, he did his best to type it in from memory. Unfortunately, he missed one letter, and his note was directed instead to an elderly preacher's wife, whose husband had passed away only the day before.

When the grieving widow checked her e-mail, she took one look at the monitor, let out a piercing scream, and fell to the floor in a dead faint. At the sound, her family rushed into the room and saw this note on the screen:

Dearest Wife,

Just got checked in. Everything prepared for your arrival tomorrow.

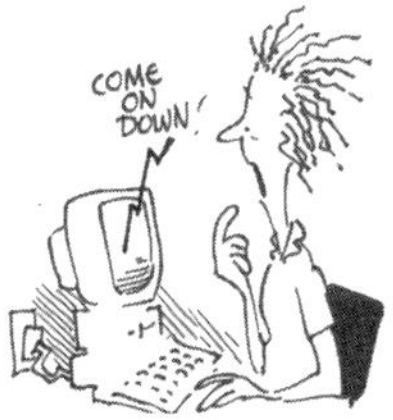

P.S. Sure is hot down here.

(www.jokebuddha.com)

Can I Have Fries With That Order?

A physician was driving her four-year-old daughter to preschool. The doctor had left her stethoscope on the car seat, and her little girl picked it up and began playing with it.

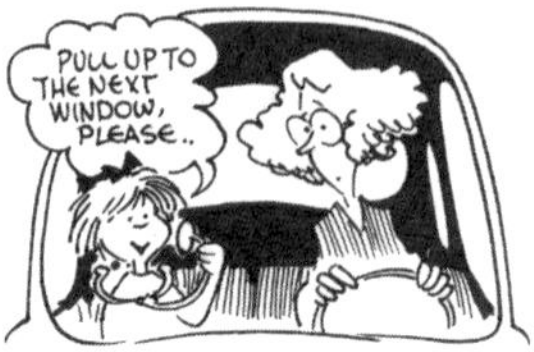

"Be still, my heart," thought the doctor. "My daughter wants to walk in my footsteps!"

Then the child spoke into the instrument.

"Welcome to McDonald's. May I take your order?"

(Kids Say the Funniest Things, submitted by Qiltmeister)

* * * * *

Blame It On the Cost of Healthcare!

Federal and most states' laws require that prisoners be furnished with adequate medical care. But Larry Causey sought benefits of the law more deliberately than most previous inmates. He pled guilty after being arrested in his car outside the post office in West Monroe, LA, which he had just held up. He apparently held the robbery for the sole purpose of being incarcerated so his cancer could be treated.

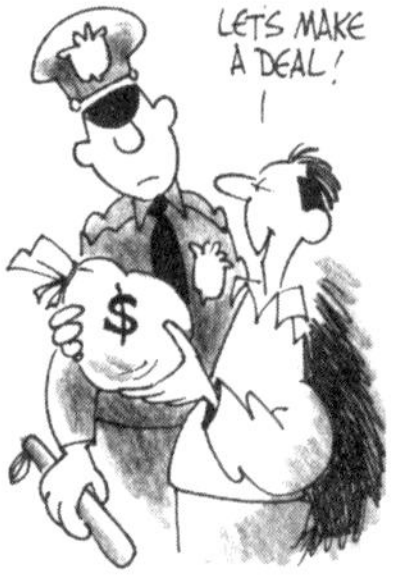

Upon being jailed, Causey was immediately prescribed three drugs and scheduled for a colonoscopy.

Seems an elderly gentleman had serious hearing problems for a number of years. He went to the doctor, and the doctor was able to have him fitted for a set of hearing aids that allowed the gentleman to hear 100%.

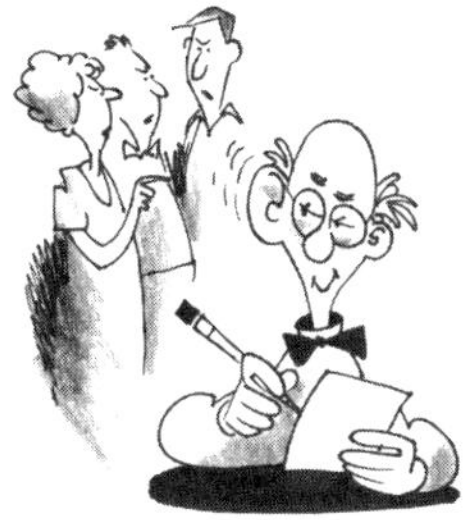

The elderly gentleman went back in a month to the doctor, and the doctor said, "Your hearing is perfect. Your family must be really pleased that you can hear again." To which the gentleman replied, "Oh, I haven't told my family yet. I just sit around and listen to the conversations. I've changed my will three times already!"

(www.jokesbite.com)

* * * * *

Watch Out for Those MRIs!

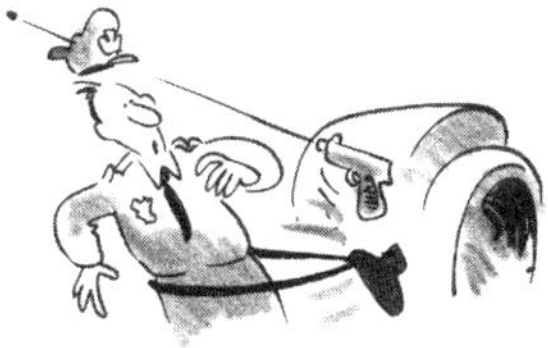

An off-duty police officer reporting for an MRI while armed had the super-powerful magnet suck his gun away and slam it against the machine, causing one round to fire into a wall.

NEXT!

The man looked a little worried when the doctor came in to administer his annual physical, so the first thing the doctor did was to ask whether anything was troubling him.

"Well, to tell the truth, Doc, yes," answered the patient. "You see, I seem to be getting forgetful. No, it's actually worse than that. I'm never sure I can remember where I put the car, or whether I answered a letter, or where I'm going, or what it is I'm going to do once I get there—if I get there. So, I really need your help. What can I do?"

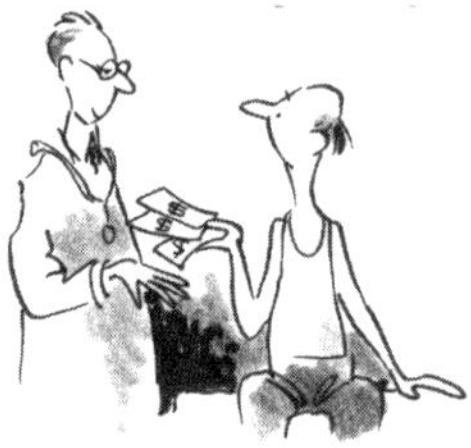

The doctor mused for a moment, then answered in his kindest tone, "Pay me in advance!"

(www.medical-jokes.com)

* * * * *

"No need for me to come out to the house," the doctor told the old woman. "I've checked my files and your husband isn't really ill at all. He just thinks he's sick."

A week later, the doctor telephoned to make sure his diagnosis had been correct. "How's your hubby today?" he asked.

"Worse," replied the woman. "Now he thinks he's dead."

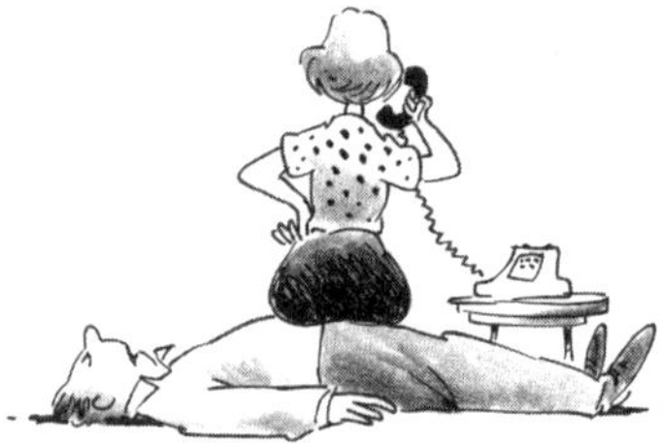

A man returns from the doctor and tells his wife that his doctor told him he has only 24 hours to live. Given this prognosis, the man asks his wife for some affection. Naturally, she agrees, and they make whoopee.

About six hours later, the husband approaches his wife and says, "Honey, you know I now have only 18 hours to live. Could we please do it one more time?" Of course, the wife agrees, and they do it again.

Later, as the man gets into bed, he looks at his watch and realizes that now he has only 8 hours left. He touches his wife's shoulder, and asks, "Honey, please … just one more time before I die." She says, "Of course, Dear," and they make love for the third time.

After this session, the wife rolls over and falls asleep. The man, however, worried about his impending death, tosses and turns, until he's down to 4 more hours. He taps his wife, who rouses. "Honey, I have only 4 more hours. Do you think we could …"

At this point, the wife sits up and says, "Listen, I have to get up in the morning. You don't!"

* * * * *

May I Leave on My Socks and Shoes?

According to an article in the *Journal of General Internal Medicine*, it takes physicians just as long to examine patients who wear gowns as it does to examine those who choose to stay dressed. What's more, the time it takes to undress, put on a gown, and get dressed again adds an extra four minutes, on average, to the time already spent in the examination room.

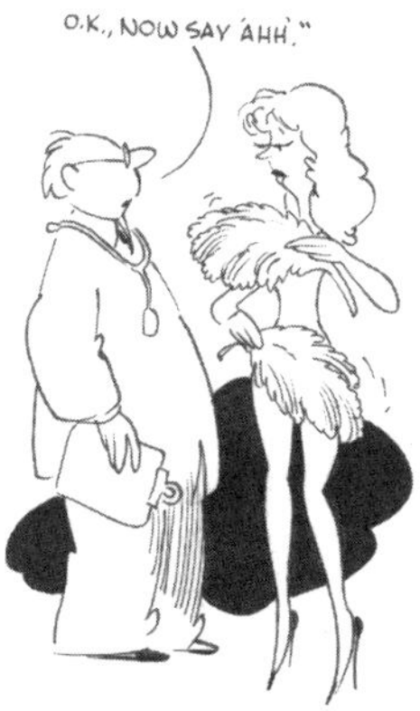

It's All in My Head!

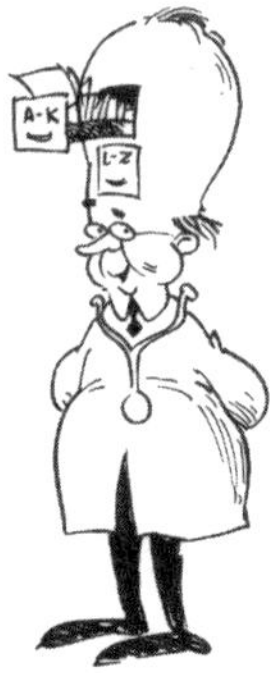

The Arkansas State Medical Board ordered Jewel Byron Grimmett, Jr., a family physician in Waldo, to start keeping written records. At a hearing, Grimmett told board members that he has kept all patient histories, including prescription records, only in his head for the 35 years he had practiced medicine. Grimmett avoided license revocation: he was Waldo's only doctor.

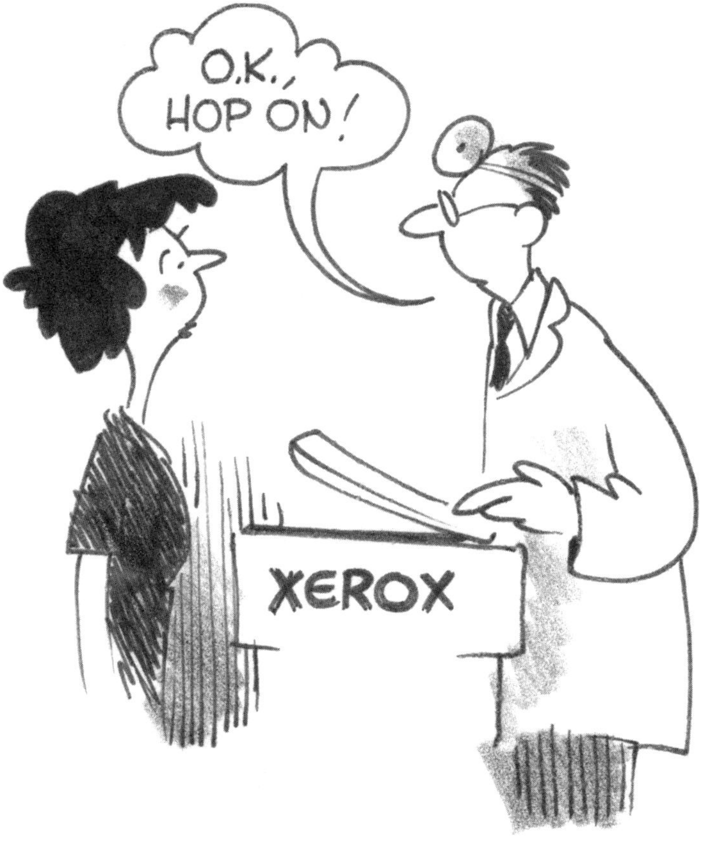
O.K.,
HOP ON!
XEROX

Chapter 10: The Grinning Reaper

"Laughter may not always add years to your life, but it will add life to your years."

– I.B. Wright

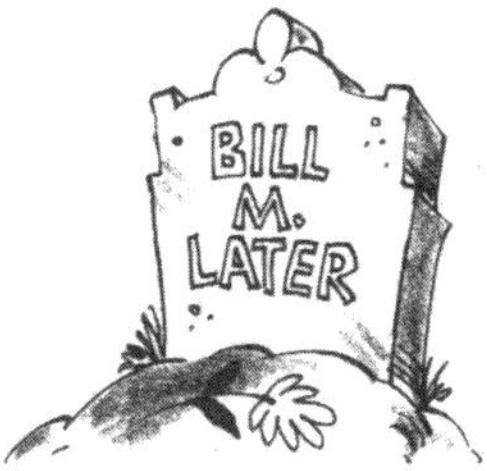

I was told I had six months to live when I was diagnosed with cancer. That was over 17 years ago now. But I never was a good listener.

Certainly death is one of the first things people think about when they hear the words, "You have cancer." And I thought about it, too.

But I did make a decision that no matter how many days, months, or years I had, that I wanted to live every day to its fullest. Bob Hope once said, "When you get over 95, every day is your day." And I made a vow to laugh every single day. One of my dear friends and fellow authors Allen Klein, author of *The Healing Power of Humor, The Courage to Laugh: Humor in the Face of Death* and his newest book, *Learning to Laugh When you Feel Like Crying: Embracing Life After Loss,* had this to say when I spoke with him:

I call myself a "Jollytologist." This unusual career began shortly after my wife died as a result of primary biliary serosis—a rare liver disease. I started to explore the value of humor because of the important role it played before, during, and after her death.

At first, it seemed strange to me that my career in humor would emerge out of a loss. But as I began to work in the death and dying field, it seemed less bizarre.

After investigating humor's benefits for dozens of years now and frequently seeing how humor helps lift people's spirits during a loss, I am no longer surprised by the connection between humor and death.

Certainly illnesses such as cancer or AIDS may not be what we think of as laughing matter. They, after all, often involve pain and the loss of life or limb. Still, life goes on, and funny things happen in spite of illness and death.

Christine Clifford is a great example of a patient who is taking care of friends and family with humor. Here, too, is something which I have observed again and again—many people don't know why, but they are drawn toward humor in tough times. On one level, we brush off comedy as being trivial, merely something to make us laugh. But on a deeper, perhaps unconscious level, we know how powerful a good laugh can be.

*****

A dear friend of mine, Joe Tye from Iowa wrote a beautiful poem that I've always treasured. It goes like this:

I Cheated Death

I cheated death when I visited a friend who was dying in the hospital
rather than worrying about who would visit me when I was in that bed.

I cheated death when I ...

Walked through the garden and cut a fresh rose.
Went to the church and donated old clothes.
Felt the spring clover run through my toes.
Snuggled a kitty with the tip of my nose.

I cheated death when my heart was full of woe and despair, and I picked
up my pen and wrote a poem of joy and hope.

I cheated death when I ...

Re-read *The Prophet* with a cup of hot tea.

Remembered warm breezes from a tropical sea.

Cooed at a baby who smiled back at me.

Went into the woods and planted a tree.

I cheated death when I stopped agonizing about all the yesterdays than never were and all the tomorrows that will never be and was simply grateful for all the todays that always are.

I cheated death when I ...

Listened to Mozart while I counted the stars.

Spread old-fashioned jelly from old-fashioned jars.

Stayed up late and watched Venus loves Mars.

Escaped one last time from fear's prison bars.

I cheated death when I looked up at the empty cross over the altar and remembered the promise that someday my cross will be empty as well.

I cheated death when I ...

Accepted that things don't always turn out my way.

Noticed small miracles that happen each day.

Invited a lost soul to come in and stay.

Learned to not worry but rather to pray.

Alas, my friends, we all have to go sometime. So when we do, I certainly hope we can do so with a good sense of humor. After all ... the funeral industry has certainly chosen to do so.

Funeral directors make me laugh. They don't mean to. They just can't help it.

As evidence, do what I did twelve summers ago and drive through Arlington, Texas, and eventually you will come upon a bright white billboard advertising a local funeral home—one that prides itself on its attention to detail, apparently, but that carries inexpensive products.

"*Boxwell Brothers*" it reads.

"It's a joke?" I asked my host, seated next to me in her red Taurus. "No, they've been around for years. Done real well."

The next spring I was in the town of my golfing dreams, Augusta, Georgia. Driving back after spending a balmy Thursday at the Masters Tournament, I noticed alongside the road a small French restaurant. I stepped in, took one of the eight dark oak tables, and was treated to some tender salmon and a glass of Chardonnay. A sense of *déjà vu* came over me, and was justified when I walked out of the restaurant, adjusted my eyes to the darkness, and spotted a billboard for yet another funeral home.

"Caskets and MORE." Why the glee? I thought. And what more *could* there be? Cone-shaped party hats and noisemakers for the funeral? Maybe a frequent dier's program? Wait, did they forget to add their slogan?

"We put the *fun* back in *funeral!*"

That fall I was in upstate New York walking with an old friend, recalling favorite stories on a brisk October evening, walking off a shared bottle of wine. We rounded a corner and came upon another funeral home, but reading the sign, I suspected the wine had clouded my vision. After blinking and reading the sign again, it was unmistakable. Perhaps the owners heard from one of the customers, who wanted to be sure their services had worked.

"Amigone" it read. I assume they gave that customer his money back—that, or a final blow to the head. It turns out that Amigone is actually a *chain*—there are dozens of Amigones all across New York.

Later that winter, driving east from Minneapolis to St. Paul on a freeway I'd driven every week for nine years, I once again noticed the Brown Wilburt Vaults sign, but realized I'd always sped by too quickly to notice their catchy slogan, which only compounded the irony:

Drive Safely. We Can Wait.

I once stayed overnight in a Wisconsin town where the Wagner's Funeral Home is next door to a health food store. Seemed smart to me; if the healthy food fails you, you're right there—kind of one-stop shopping.

I have a photograph—I have photographs of all these signs—but don't recall the town that claims one of the most-aptly named funeral homes ever.

It's called *Cease.*

Drive through Hot Spring, Arkansas and you'll pass by *Graves Mini Storage.* I've heard about people who store strange things, but I don't think I want to know.

One day I made a wrong turn in northern Minnesota and found myself on Cemetery Road. Nothing strange about that—there are lots of cemetery roads. But just in case the drivers weren't clear what it meant, there was another sign right below that.

"No Exit."

Those funny Minnesotans are topped only by the Oregonians near the town of Nehalem whose Cemetery Road sign warns drivers, if they didn't know already:

"Dead end."

Of course, funeral directors are laughing these days. What other business has such guaranteed demand? Not everyone uses gel pens or dental floss—in parts of England, it appears they don't use toothbrushes, either. But everyone—except Dick Clark, apparently—dies.

The funeral directors are especially cheery these days, because we baby boomers are getting older. I know directors and their glee because I attended one of their national events and noticed their happy theme:

"Ohio Funeral Directors Association. Building for the Future."

Having spoken at over three hundred similar meetings, I know there is a popular expert on demographics who tours the funeral business circuit with a beloved PowerPoint presentation, which shows how baby boomers are edging closer to death. He gets standing ovations wherever he goes, even from the directors in their late 70s who, as usual, are oblivious to the irony of it all, too intoxicated by the presentation's first and final slide:

"Boom Days Ahead for Death!"

But good for all of them for putting the fun back in funeral, because that's what I'm planning, too. I'm thinking about asking Ellen DeGeneres to host and asking my kids to place Whoopee cushions on all the pews.

Some people say they'll drag their feet right to Heaven's Gate. I have a better plan. I'm heading there on a pogo stick, laughing all the way.

Have You Heard (Resources for People with Cancer)

About … Organizations?

The following organizations can provide valuable information to you about cancer:

www.cancer.org is the official website for the American Cancer Society, providing information, support and more. (800)227–2345

www.chemo101.com is your one-stop resource for essential, accurate, and objective information to make the best health and financial decisions to attain the maximum benefits of chemotherapy. (612)845–8769

www.caringbridge.org/cancer is Caring Bridge, which creates free personal, private websites that provide support for cancer during treatment, recovery, and beyond. (651)452–7940

www.cancer.gov The National Cancer Institute coordinates the National Cancer Program, which conducts and supports research, training, health information dissemination, and other programs with respect to the cause, diagnosis, prevention, and treatment of cancer, rehabilitation from cancer, and the continuing care of cancer patients and their families. (800)4-CANCER

www.cancerhopenetwork.org is the Cancer Hope Network and provides free and confidential one-on-one support to cancer patients and their families. (800)552–4366

www.cancersupportcommunity.org is the Cancer Support Community, a non-profit dedicated to ensuring that all people affected by cancer are empowered by knowledge, strengthened by action, and sustained by community. (202)659–9709

www.livestrong.org/CancerSupport fights to improve the lives of people affected by cancer by providing free, confidential one-on-one support to anyone affected by cancer. (855)220–7777

www.canceradvocacy.org is the National Coalition for Cancer Survivorship. To combat the isolation many people fee after being diagnosed, this group offers information about treatment, employment, and insurance issues, as well as emotional support. (888)937–6227

About … Books?

Tears of Joy: In Sickness and in Health a Cancer Survivor and Their Caregiver Share Their Story by Jerry Hanks and Bobbi de Cordova-Hanks. $12.95 (877)BUY-BOOK, or **www.speakersforlife.com**

The BEST NEWS about Radiation Therapy: How to Cope & Survive by Carol L. Kornmehl, MD, FACRO. $14.95 (800)462–6420, or **www.RT-SupportDoc.com**

Challenge Cancer and Win! Step-by-Step Nutrition Action Plans for Your Specific Cancer by Kim Dalzell, PhD, RD, LD. $22.95 (800)832–2983, or **www.challengecancerandwin.com**

Caregiving without Regrets: 3 Steps to Avoid Burnout and Manage Disappointment, Guilt and Anger by Vicki Rackner, MD. $14.95 (425)451–3777, or **www.DrVicki.org**

Laughter, Tears, Silence: Expressive Meditations to Calm Your Mind and Open Your Heart by Pragito Dove. $14.95 (415)884–2100, or **www.pragito.com**

Rays of Hope In Times of Loss: Courage and Comfort for Grieving Hearts by Susan Zimmerman, LMFT, ChFC. $18.95 (800)525–5301, or **www.ahaplan.com**

About … Resources for Children?

Believe in Tomorrow Children's Foundation is a national non-profit organization that provides ongoing services that bring comfort, joy, and hope to critically ill children and their families including Retreat and Hospital Housing, Hands On Adventures, and Pain Management & Distraction. (800)933–5470, or **www.believeintomorrow.org**

www.LocksOfLove.org is a public, non-profit organization that provides hairpieces to financially disadvantaged children in the United States and Canada under age 21 suffering from long-term medical hair loss from any diagnosis. (888)896–1588.

CURE Childhood Cancer is a non-profit organization dedicated to conquering childhood cancer through research, education, patient, and family support. (800)443-CURE, or **www.curechildhoodcancer.org**

Kids Konnected provides support for children ages 3–18 who have a parent with cancer. Call (800)899–2866, or **www.kidskonnected.org**

Home Care for Seriously Ill Children: A Manual for Parents prepared by D. Gay Holdow, RN, MSW and Ida M. Martinson, RN, PhD, FANN. Distributed by Children's Hospice International. $18.00 (703)684–0330, or **www.CHIonline.org**

About … Products?

One Move at a Time: Exercise for Women Recovering from Breast Cancer Surgery is a DVD with gentle exercises to get you back in motion. $19.95 (952)944–0639 or visit **www.CancerClub.com** for this and many other cancer gift items including ornaments, custom jewelry, stuffed animals and more! Don't forget to laugh! ™

Laughter: Prescription for a Cure! is a DVD featuring author Christine Clifford in a one-hour presentation, sharing the hysterical stories and inspirational events that have tickled the funny bones of audiences all over the world. $19.94 (952)944–0639, or **www.CancerClub.com** Don't forget to laugh! ™

Headwear etc. provides head covers, bandanas, wigs, hats, and more at Marilyn Robinson's online boutique. Visit **www.headwearetc.com** or email **Marilyn@headwearetc.com**

About … Services?

Air Charity Network is a non-profit group of volunteer pilots who provide free air transportation anywhere in the U.S. to financially strapped patients who qualify. For information, call (877) 621–7177, or **www.aircharitynetwork.org**

Cancer Answer is a phone line with a cancer clinical nurse specialist available Monday to Friday, 8:30am- 4:30pm EST to answer cancer-related questions or requests for clarification. Provided by the Cleveland Clinic Taussig Cancer Center. Call (800)862–7798, or visit **www.clevelandclinic.org/cancer**

Coping with Cancer is a magazine for people whose lives have been touched by cancer. Now in its 25th year of service. (615)790–2400, or **www.copingmag.com**

Dream Foundation grants wishes to adults 18 years and older whose life expectancy is less than one year, and whose limited resources leave them unable to manifest their dreams. (805)564–2131, or **www.dreamfoundation.org** and help a dream come true!

Vital Options International TeleSupport Cancer Network facilitates a global cancer dialogue, through *The Group Room*®, a call-in radio cancer show that allows people from all walks of life to meet, talk, teach, learn, and share information. Visit **www.vitaloptions.org**

World's Leading Authorities on the Use of Therapeutic Humor

Patty Wooten

Patty Wooten is a nurse-humorist, and a woman who knows how to laugh at life. She is a veteran of countless radio and television shows, and her work has been featured in *USA Today*, *Better Homes & Gardens*, *Psychology Today*, and *USA Weekend* magazine. She is the author of two books, *Heart, Humor and Healing* and *Compassionate Laughter*. As an international speaker and past President of the Association for Applied and Therapeutic Humor, Patty has tickled the funny bones of over 100,000 happy people. In 2002, Patty was the recipient of the Lifetime Achievement Award from the Association for Applied and Therapeutic Humor. She is President of Jest for The Health of It.

To reach Patty, call (831)425–8436 or email her at
PWooten@JestHealth.com

www.JestHealth.com

Dr. Cliff Kuhn

Dr. Clifford Kuhn is a 45-year practicing psychiatrist, medical school professor, and internationally acclaimed humor expert who has helped thousands unleash the power of humor to become healthier, happier, and more successful. He offers workshops and keynotes based on his patented "HA HA HA Prescription." His latest book, *It All Starts With a Smile: Seven Steps to Being Happier Right Now*, has been described by one reviewer as "the best how-to book on humor I have ever read."

To reach Dr. Kuhn, call (502)722–8732 or email him at
DoctorLaugh@aol.com

www.DrCliffordKuhn.com

Vicki Woodyard

Vicki Woodyard is a writer who lives in Atlanta, Georgia. Her book, *Life With a Hole In It: That's How The Light Gets In,* tells her story. Her late husband Bob died of multiple myeloma in 2004, and they lost their only daughter to a fatal form of childhood cancer when she was seven. "Cherish your loved ones and cherish laughter as the spiritual gift that it is." Vicki has written jokes for Joan Rivers, Jay Leno, Jeff Foxworthy, and more.

To reach Vicki, email her at **VW9633@gmail.com**

www.VickiWoodyard.com

Gavin Jerome

Gavin Jerome has been a stand-up comedian and professional entertainer for over twenty years. He has worked with Jerry Seinfeld, Paul Reiser, Dennis Miller, Steve Harvey, and Pat Paulson. For over a decade, Gavin has been providing humor workshops for companies worldwide. His programs are fun, funny, and filled with valuable content to help companies and individuals reduce stress, enjoy work more, and want to strangle co-workers less. He is the author of *Gavin Jerome's Comedy College How-to-Handbook,* now in its eighth printing.

To reach Gavin, call (800)96-GAVIN or email him at
MoraleMechanic@mchsi.com

www.MoraleMechanic.com

Mark Darby

Mark Darby, RN, is the author of several books and articles on humor including *Reflections on the Hands of a Nurse.* He is currently writing a novel about healthcare based on the story of the nurse midwives in Exodus, Chapter Two due out in 2012.

To reach Mark, call (402)451–3459 or email him at
MarkDarby@MDarby.com

www.MDarby.com

Dr. Edward Dunkelblau

Dr. Edward Dunkelblau is an Illinois Licensed Psychologist and the Director of the Institute for Emotionally Intelligent Learning. He is an internationally known speaker and consultant on the topics of social emotional learning, organizational change issues, team building, and on the applications of humor in business, healthcare, and education. He is a contributing author to the *Handbook of Humor and Psychotherapy* and *Humor and Wellness in Clinical Intervention.*

His work has been featured in the *New York Times, Chicago Tribune, USA Today, Chicago Parent,* on NPR, *CNN Live* and he was co-host on an episode of the Emmy award-winning TV show NICK NEWS with Linda Ellerbee. Dr. Dunkelblau has been awarded the Alumni of the Year Award from Kansas University School of Education and the Distinguished Alumni Award from Columbia University Teachers College.

To reach Ed, call (847)803–6166 or email him at **DrLaugh01@aol.com**

www.TeachEQ.com

Izzy Gesell

Izzy Gesell is "America's Humorologist" and Head Honcho at IzzyG & Company. He is the author of *Cancer and the Healing Power of Play* and *Playing Along: Group Learning Activities Borrowed from Improvisation Theater*. As a keynote speaker and group facilitator, Izzy has helped hundreds of organizations and corporations reap the benefits of an active sense of humor.

To reach Izzy, call (413)586–2634 or email him at **Izzy@IzzyG.com**

www.IzzyG.com Blog: **www.PracticedSpontaneity.com**

Ann E. Weeks

Ann E. Weeks, DNS, RN is a nationally known speaker, author of seven books and numerous stories. To help you access a week's worth of humor via email, let Ann add you to her weekly eNewsletter entitled "WEEKS OF FUN." It contains a healing tip, jest tip, creativity tip, juicy tidbits, and much more!

To reach Ann, call (502)458–2461 or email her at
AnnWeeks@insightbb.com
www.DrAnnWeeks.net

Allen Klein, MA, CSP

Allen Klein is a former director of The Life-Death Transitions Institute in San Francisco. Currently he is an award-winning professional speaker and best-selling author. Klein is a recipient of a Lifetime Achievement Award from the Association for Applied and Therapeutic Humor, a Certified Speaking Professional with the National Speakers Association, and an inductee in the Hunter College, New York City, Hall of Fame. Klein is the author of 17 books including *The Healing Power of Humor, The Courage to Laugh,* and his latest book *Learning to Laugh When You Feel Like Crying: Embracing Life After Loss.*

Humor@AllenKlein.com

www.AllenKlein.com

About the Author

All of us have read or heard stories about people who turn lemons into lemonade. It isn't often that we get the privilege of meeting such an individual.

Before her bout with breast cancer, **Christine Clifford** had definitely cracked the "glass ceiling." By age 40, she was Senior Executive Vice President for The SPAR Group, an international marketing firm in New York. Once the top salesperson in the multi-billion dollar retail services industry, Christine's accounts included Kmart, Toys "R" Us, Procter & Gamble, AT&T, Mattel Toys, and Revlon.

Diagnosed with breast cancer in December of 1994, Christine wrote six award-winning portrayals of her story in her books entitled *Not Now ...I'm Having a No Hair Day!*, *Our Family Has Cancer, Too!* written especially for children, *Inspiring Breakthrough Secrets to Live Your Dreams*, *Cancer Has Its Privileges: Stories of Hope and Laughter*, *Your Guardian Angel's Gift*, *You, Inc. The Art of Selling Yourself*, and Christine's newest book *The Clue Phone's Ringing ... It's for You! Healing Humor for Women Divorcing* (Anshan, 2011).

Christine is President and CEO of The Cancer Club®, the world's largest producer of humorous and helpful products for people with cancer. She owns an anti-aging distributorship (**www.LifeVantage.com/liveyoung**), and is CEO of Divorcing Divas® (**www.DivorcingDivas.net**), and Christine Clifford Enterprises (**www.christineclifford.com**).

Featured in over 2,000 media hits, Christine appeared on *CNN Live* as "one of the world's leading authorities on the use of therapeutic humor."

Host of *The Christine Clifford Celebrity Golf Tournament*, Christine's inaugural event in 1998 raised over $100,000, making it the most successful first-year event in the history of the American Cancer Society. Christine's contribution has been over $1,000,000.

Christine earned her CSP designation (Certified Speaking Professional) from the National Speakers Association. Fewer than 550 people hold the CSP, putting Christine in the top 7% of professional speakers worldwide.

She has two sons, Tim & Brooks, and is Grandmother to Siberian Husky Skylar in Minneapolis.

About the Illustrator 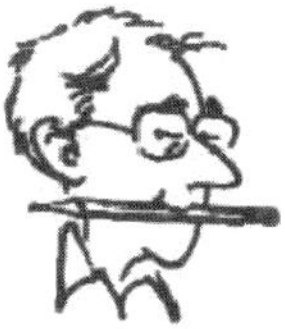

A native Minnesotan, **Jack Lindstrom** specializes in humorous illustrations for various print media—books, periodicals, and newspapers. For many years, he collaborated with William Wells to produce a daily comic strip, *Bull 'N' Bears* for United Feature Syndicate. He is also a partner in Finkstrom Productions specializing in greeting cards and humorous calendars.

Jack is married to his high school sweetheart, receives unsolicited advice from two grown children, and helps to spoil his three grandchildren whenever the opportunity presents itself … which is often.

About The Cancer Club®

"A shared gift of laughter is a priceless gift to the spirit."

– Christine Clifford

The Cancer Club, based in Minneapolis, Minnesota, was created by Christine Clifford in 1995 in response to her experience with breast cancer. Christine, whose mother died of breast cancer at the age of forty-two, found that during her own treatment, family and friends were supportive, but they also were careful to avoid humorous conversation or topics around her.

Needing a lift, Christine began to search for signs of humor in herself and her predicament. She found them daily. The more she laughed, the stronger she grew, and The Cancer Club® was born.

The critically acclaimed Cancer Club® is the first organization to offer hope and support to cancer patients, their families and friends through the healing power of humor. It serves as an international clearinghouse for people affected by cancer, offering inspirational gifts and providing information and resources through their website, www.cancerclub.com.

Cancer Club® products include all of Christine's books, including *Not Now … I'm Having a No Hair Day!*, *Our Family Has Cancer, Too!* (written especially for children), *Cancer Has Its Privileges: Stories of Hope & Laughter, Inspiring Breakthrough Secrets to Live Your Dreams, Your Guardian Angel's Gift*, DVDs, custom jewelry, stuffed animals, ornaments, and more. A special DVD, *One Move at a Time! Exercise for Women Recovering from Breast Cancer Surgery*, was written, directed and produced by Christine Clifford.

Christine Clifford is president and chief executive officer of The Cancer Club®. As a member of the National Speakers Association and a Certified

Speaking Professional, Christine lectures and tours on behalf of many organizations internationally and is happy to share her stories of using humor to get through life's adversities with you and your organization.

For more information about The Cancer Club®, call (952)944-0639. Email us at: Christine@cancerclub.com. Or write:

The Cancer Club®
PO Box 24747
Edina, MN 55424-0747

www.cancerclub.com

Don't forget to laugh! ™

Other Books by Christine Clifford

Not Now … I'm Having a No Hair Day: Humor & Healing for People with Cancer

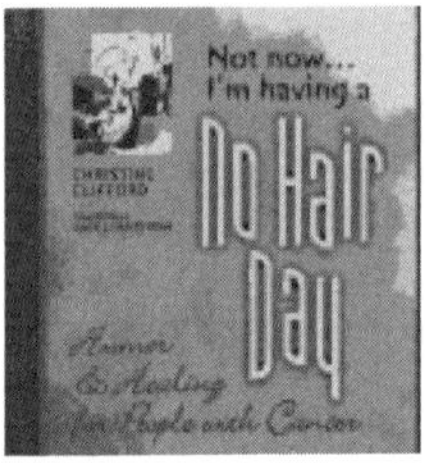

Written by Christine Clifford
Illustrated by Jack Lindstrom
112 pages
ISBN 1-57025-120-7
Publication Date: August 1, 1996 (University of Minnesota Press)

Inspired by the author's experience with breast cancer, *Not Now … I'm Having a No Hair Day!* is the first book of its kind to offer hope to cancer patients, their families and friends through the healing power of humor.

In her straightforward style, first-time author Christine Clifford, CSP paints a realistic picture of what it's like discover cancer, undergo surgery, and endure radiation and chemotherapy treatments. But unlike most cancer patients, she manages to find humor in herself and her predicament. Throughout the book, her moments of fear, frustration, uncertainty, love, and joy are captured by the gentle wit of illustrator Jack Lindstrom in 60 cartoons that reveal the vulnerability and strength of the human soul. Together, Clifford and Lindstrom show readers how the power of laughter and positive thinking go a long way toward promoting recovery and growth.

"… No Hair Day! is a wonderful book. Humor, that's the most important ingredient for facing the enemy–cancer. I had breast cancer in 1979–surgery, chemotherapy for a year. I'm sure it was laughter from God that saved me."
- Julie Harris, star of stage, screen, and television.

"I've always felt that humor is even better than chicken soup for the healing process. My friend Christine Clifford's book handles grave subject matter with sensitivity and warmth."
- Jim Davis, cartoonist and creator of Garfield™

"You are doing great work. I am inspired by your message."
- Jack Canfield, author of *Chicken Soup for the Soul*

Our Family Has Cancer, Too!

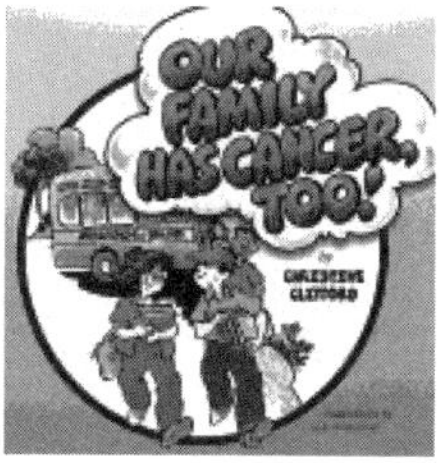

Written by Christine Clifford
Illustrated by Jack Lindstrom
64 pages
ISBN 1-57025-144-4
Publication Date: October 1997 (University of Minnesota Press)

Christine has broken new ground once again with this book. With the help and insight of her son, Tim, Christine has explored the issues facing families when cancer becomes a part of life.

Author's Note to Children
Cancer isn't fair, but through it all, know you are loved … and that you can help your family because you bring a special piece to the puzzle … You!

Author's Note to Parents
When I was first diagnosed with cancer, I decided that in my family we would not waste any of the time we had together. I hope this book will encourage you to talk about the disease—but most of all, to truly live.

Complete with a glossary for children, Christine's book offers an opportunity for you and your family to learn and share feelings with each other about cancer and to answer the questions most kids have:
- What is cancer?
- What changes will happen to our family?
- What are the treatments like?
- How long will it take to get through the cancer experience?
- What do I tell my friends?

But most importantly, it teaches you how to laugh together! Once again, Clifford and Lindstrom show readers how the power of laughter and positive thinking go a long way toward promoting recovery and growth.

Cancer Has Its Privileges: Stories of Hope and Laughter

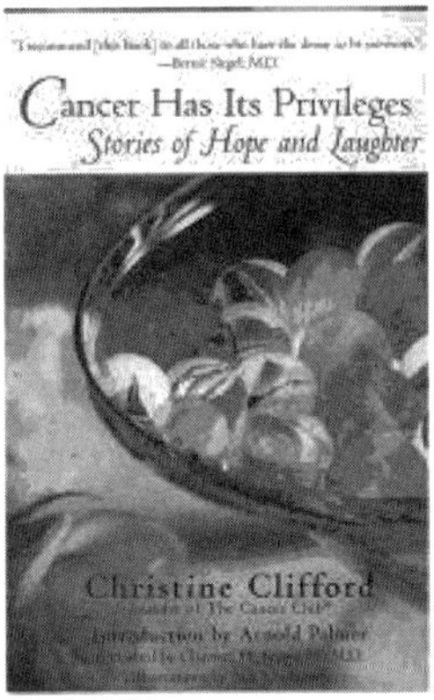

Written by Christine Clifford
160 pages
ISBN 0-399-52776-1
Publication Date: May 2002 (Perigee)

Cancer survivor and founder of The Cancer Club®, Christine Clifford, CSP has been sharing her inspiring, humorous outlook on living with cancer with thousands of cancer patients and their families. Now she has gathered a collection of battlefield stories and anecdotes from her fellow survivors that go from the outright hilarious to the downright moving, and combined them with her own personal story of triumphant survival.

"A remarkable woman whose sense of humor became her best weapon against an often dehumanizing disease."
- Arnold Palmer, from the Introduction

"A book filled with what I call survival behavior. A meaningful life is built on love and laughter and this book shares both ... I recommend it to all those who have the desire to be survivors."
- Bernie Siegel, M.D., author of *Love, Medicine and Miracles*

"The perfect dose of medicine for anyone whose life has been touched by cancer."
- Michele Smith, Olympic gold medalist

"You don't have to have had cancer to be a survivor. Christine's inspirational and pathologically positive attitude should be shared by everyone who has faced adversity. God definitely has a plan for this woman."
-Larry Gatlin, Grammy Award winning singer/songwriter

Your Guardian Angel's Gift

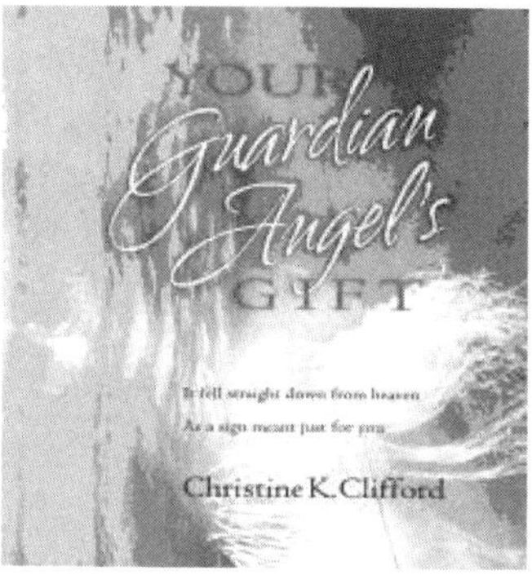

Written by Christine Clifford
64 pages
ISBN 1-932458-30-1
Publication Date: August 1, 2005 (Bronze Bow Publishing)

You or someone you love, now or very soon, needs the message this book contains. As the title says, it is a gift. Almost all of us can remember the time, date, and place we were when we learned that we or someone we care about received bad news. Negative emotions filled our heads, feelings of denial, grief, anger, and fear. Following the initial shock, we turn to the one thing that makes us human—our will to survive, and then thrive.

Your Guardian Angel's Gift, a beautiful full-color gift book, is the perfect answer to this need. It has an unforgettable message of hope and encouragement that transcends life's challenges and goes straight to the heart of anyone facing adversity. After all, we all have a Guardian Angel up in heaven. Yours has sent a feather to the ground to let you know she's watching over you.

Inspiring Breakthrough Secrets to Live Your Dreams

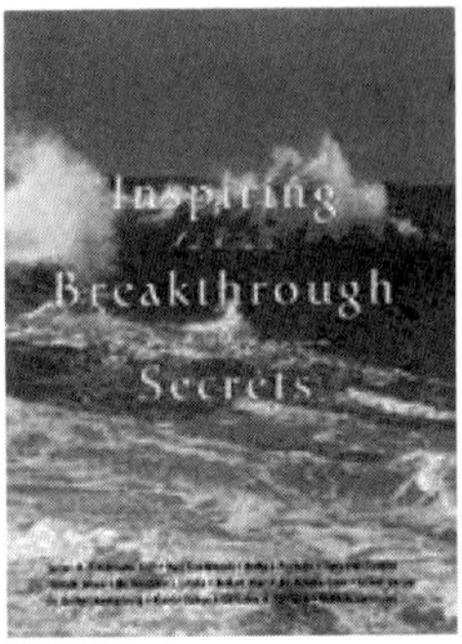

Co-Authored by Christine Clifford
224 pages
ISBN 1-890427-08-X
Publication Date: October 1, 2001

From the award-winning author of *Not Now … I'm Having a No Hair Day!* and *Our Family Has Cancer, Too!* comes a book that will transform you to take action to live the life you've always dreamed of.
"If you believe in yourself, your product, your service, or your cause, anything is possible."
- Christine Clifford

North America's most inspiring authorities in personal and professional transformation reveal secrets, insights, and strategies that will empower you to break through your limitations and live your dreams.
In her straightforward style, author, Professional Speaker and President/CEO of The Cancer Club, Christine Clifford, CSP believes adversity can be the stepping-stone to living your dream. In the chapter, "The Blessings of Misfortune: Learn to Spin Straw into Gold," Christine will lead you through the steps that will help your dreams come true.

"Everyone wants to have a breakthrough now. This master teacher has, at long last, congealed her genius in this book. You can create phenomenal breakthroughs. Read it! Use it! Share it! And make your life a masterpiece."
- Mark Victor Hanson, co-creator, #1 *New York Times* best-selling series *Chicken Soup for the Soul*

"Here it is! This inspiring book is warm, witty and a wonderful way to clarify your heart's desire. If you follow its practical ideas, your whole life opens up before you like a summer sunrise."
- Brian Tracy, Author, *The 100 Absolutely Unbreakable Laws of Business Success*